CW00972897

My Secret Life

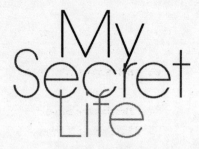

My Secret Life

SEXUAL REVELATIONS
FROM LONG-TERM LOVERS

Brigid McConville

Thorsons
An Imprint of HarperCollins*Publishers*

Thorsons
An Imprint of HarperCollins*Publishers*
77–85 Fulham Palace Road
Hammersmith, London W6 8JB

Published by Thorsons 1998
1 3 5 7 9 10 8 6 4 2

A catalogue record for this book is available
from the British Library

ISBN 0 7225 3662 3

Printed by Caledonian International Book Manufacturing Ltd, Glasgow

Contents

ACKNOWLEDGEMENTS

The list of women and men who contributed their stories to this book is long and I am extremely grateful to them all. Their names have been changed because these are otherwise 'secret lives' but I hope they will enjoy reading their own stories – while guessing who the others might belong to!

My editor, Belinda Budge, has been as positive and helpful as ever, as has Michele Turney, who polished up the final manuscript. Julia Cole, Jane Hawksley and Denise Knowles have given me the benefit of their long experience as counsellors with Relate, while my partner John Shearlaw has managed to survive a year of wondering what *exactly* I was writing about…

Many thanks to you all.

Introduction

'What's it about then?' friends would ask me as this book began to take shape. When I replied that it was about sex in long-term relationships their responses were very different:

'Hmm. That'll be a short book then!' said some, with a rueful laugh.

'Oh, that's interesting!' said others. And then, tentatively – but looking ever so slightly smug – 'You can interview me, and my man…'

All too often the first group were women with young children, struggling to reconcile the immense demands of family and paid work. The second group tended to be older women with independent children and well-established careers.

But it was useless trying to guess before an interview whether I would be hearing a tale of extended celibacy or one of extraordinary lust. I heard stories of men and women who revelled in elaborate feasts of lovemaking with their partners, and of others who felt they were condemned to a long sexual famine. I heard how some women wished their husbands would just give it a rest, while others happened to love a man who had less desire than themselves.

In the end some distinct patterns did emerge. Most of us can recognize ourselves in the tales of young women and men launching into fledgling – and often unsatisfactory – sex. Most of us have been through that first devastating love affair which provided our great sexual awakening, followed by marriage or living with someone – often the next lover down the line. Many of us know how frustrating it is when sex takes a serious nose dive after the birth of children – and stays at a low level for some time.

What encouraged me greatly was that – despite the myth that sex is for the young – it is often in their late 30s, 40s and even 50s that couples really hit their stride sexually. Only after many years of loving and living together do many of us have the confidence, experience, sensitivity – and time – truly to make the most of making love.

For good sex transcends the merely physical. It is about our relationships at the deepest level, about mind, body and spirit.

All this adds up to more than the sum of many individual experiences, because this is a remarkable time in history. Not only are we in control of our own fertility as never before, but we are also living much longer. In past centuries a 'long-term relationship' might have meant 10 or 15 years – because of short life expectancy and the toll taken by war and disease.

Today, we can expect to stay together for four times that long. Never before have people accumulated so much shared sexual experience, decades of lovemaking behind them and potentially decades ahead of them too.

This is a unique time in the history of human relationships, and this book is a unique account of what it is like to live and love at the end of the millennium.

CHAPTER I

Perspectives on Long-term Relationships

Every relationship is unique, but more or less the same issues crop up for all of us. Is sex as good as it could be – or might it be better with someone else? Does it matter if one of us goes 'off' sex, but not the other? Will desire fade with time, or does it go deeper, transforming sex into a celebration for our relationship?

Here, two couples and two individuals give insight into their secret lives.

'I love him – but our sex life is not electrifying'

Alison, 28, got together with her boyfriend, Sam, eight years ago. She is almost sure that he is right for her – but should she be concerned about the fact that she hasn't yet experienced 'explosive passion'?

'At first I enacted the role of someone very sexual but, with time, the barriers come down. It's impossible to be this sexual being over breakfast day after day for years on end. You can't play that game forever.

'Sam and I met when we were 20. We were both students in the same hall of residence and we had both played around and had lots of sexual partners before we got together. So it was a surprise to us both that it lasted.

'It has never really been electrifying between Sam and I, and until quite recently I used to wonder about meeting another man – and having that electrifying experience.'

'Young women are expected to have lots of sex.'
'I lost my virginity at 14, but it was another 10 years before I experienced orgasm. I suffered from bulimia when I was younger, and sex was a matter of boosting my self-esteem. Young women are expected to be sexy and have lots of sex. I relied on being able to attract men sexually.

'But for the first 10 years of my sex life, I never had an orgasm. And because I had my first boyfriend at 14, and then various men – and then my current relationship – I had never given myself an orgasm either.

'More recently, I've learned a bit about myself. I think orgasm is about letting go, about giving of yourself. Being aroused brings you back to some kind of primeval state, which is so much against the control and reserve women are supposed to have in our culture. We are supposed to be quiet and ladylike.'

'I told him I wanted orgasms.'

'When I had my first orgasm I realized that sex could be a completely different kind of experience. My expectations had been raised, and after that I told Sam I wanted to have orgasms when we had sex, if not always, then at least from time to time!

'Until I was comfortable with my body and with my relationship, I couldn't experience orgasm. Interestingly, my bulimia ended at about the same time that I started to have orgasms.

'With Sam I no longer have to rely on my sexuality to boost myself. I still never talk about my body because I don't want to attract attention to it, but Sam has never been critical of me or the way I look – which really helps. I feel he respects me 100 per cent.'

'I had to pretend to enjoy it.'

'But I've only recently had the confidence to talk to him about our sex life and to say – I'd like you to do it like this. I've only recently started to take steps in that direction. At first I had to pretend that it was all completely enjoyable. Because I had to be this totally sexual being.

'Then I began to ask myself – why are you playing this role when you're not getting as much out of sex as you could? Since then I've become more assertive and I've said to him that either we do it properly, or not at all. He is understanding about that.

'But generally, I'm not satisfied with the way things are in our sexual relationship, but that's partly my fault because I haven't made it a priority.'

'On week nights, I just want to go to sleep…'

'I work very hard and usually I need to go to bed by about 11 o'clock at night. More often than not there is no point in even trying to have sex during the week – unless it's a quickie – because I just want it to be over so that I can get to sleep.

'If sex is going to happen quickly, chances are that I am going to end up feeling dissatisfied. Sometimes he does get a bit frustrated, but when we do it properly it is so much better.

'When I feel I've got time, the amount of energy and enthusiasm I can put into it is 100 per cent more. Sex is so much better then than it would be in a hurry on a Sunday night. I just want to do it properly.

'My new strategy is to initiate sex sooner in the evening. It means that we can get it out of the way and it won't become an issue later.

'I'm also moving towards the idea of planning ahead to make time and set the scene a bit more. Holidays are a good time for us to get these things sorted out. We have plenty of time to talk on holiday, and time to initiate new ideas.'

'Sex is not the be all and end all.'

'I used to think sex was the be all and end all of a relationship, but I don't believe that any more. Now I feel that it's only one of a number of very important elements. Respect is very important; respecting a woman enough not to criticize her and to hold back from saying negative things.

'I have wondered if I should stay with Sam. I wonder if I should have just one night of explosive passion with another man, but I'm almost 100 per cent sure that Sam is the one to spend the rest of my life with, so our sex life is going to have to improve.'

'I've never experienced explosive passion.'

'But I wonder if either of us attaches that much importance to it. The experience of explosive passion hasn't happened in my life, and I'm coming to the conclusion that I'm just going to have to work on it with Sam. I am committed to him and I wouldn't throw away our relationship for a moment of ecstasy.

'We do it less often now than we used to, but it's better than it used to be. He'd like us to do it more often with less intensity, but for me, I need to be in a sexy mood.

'I like music, massage, setting the scene. I don't like going out for a meal before we make love; I feel very unsexy if I'm full – perhaps because of my weird relationship with food.'

'We'll have to make time to do it properly.'

'My ideal scenario is a night at home, a bottle of good wine, dim lights, some massage…But it's such a long time since it's happened like that.

'I feel that we are in a transitional phase in our relation-ship. We are going to do a lot of talking when we next go away on holiday!'

'I'm more keen to make love than he is.'

Marion, aged 35, had a series of intensely sexual relationships before she got married. Now sex is less frequent and less important – but she is happy.

'We've been together for six years and we are still very affectionate and tactile. There is a lot of gentleness, care and concern for each other. We have a lot of touching and caressing which sometimes moves on to become sexual. Our relationship is still developing.

'But I do miss the kind of heightened sexual pleasure I had in previous relationships; it would be nice to have that level of intensity – but it isn't there in our relationship. So I do have some sense of loss in terms of sexual passion, but I decided that it was worth it for the more balanced, harmonious and creative existence which we now have. This has been a healthy choice for myself.'

'In my 20s I wouldn't have made this choice…'
'In my 20s I wouldn't have made this choice. It took time and other lovers to discover what I really needed. My relationships in the past were always very passionate and dramatic – and then they were all over. Before I got married I had one roller-coaster affair which lasted for three years. It was intensely passionate, but not well founded. All my energy and thought and time went into that relationship.

'With my husband things are different – very much more reasonable and mature. He encourages who I am and what I want to do which is so refreshing after being in all-consuming relationships. Having been through those earlier experiences has certainly made things easier for me now. Our marriage is absolutely safe and totally secure. It is affection based; we are friends and should it ever end I'm sure we would remain friends.

'My husband is an artist, and I've had to get used to the fact that when he's involved in painting a picture, he just isn't sexual. I am more sexual than he is, and unless I'm really tired, I'm keen to make love.'

'I used to have good sex, but not good relationships.'

'Sex is certainly more on my mind than it is on his. But that's fine by me, because when sex is not an option, I find that my energy is freed up to do other things. In the past, sex was the focus for my energy, but now I can use this energy in my inter-actions with friends and to be more creative.

'"Passion" is something you can feel for many things – life, the earth – not just for your lover. There are many different types of ecstasy.

'In my previous relationship, the only touching of each other was sexual touching. When you have no other kind of contact, every time you make love it is highly charged. That can make for good sex, but not a very good relationship.

'I'm lucky that my husband is so tactile, because unlike couples who don't touch unless they are having sex, we don't have to rely on sex to show our love for each other. What we have is a synthesis.

'The way we deal with the difference in our libidos is most-ly through humour. We joke about the fact that I want sex and he doesn't – and that our timing is usually off. The moment inspiration strikes him for a new picture, I'm keen! Then he's finished a picture – and I'm tired!'

'I'm quite happy to masturbate.'

'I'm very happy to be with my partner and so this difference in desire is an issue that we deal with quite comfortably and positively. We talk about it a lot and he will apologize to me about being in asexual mode while I'm not. But I'm quite happy to masturbate and we work our way around the issue without rows or resentment.

'He may be preoccupied with a painting for weeks on end, which doesn't mean we don't make love for weeks, just that he is not very focused on sex. If I decide to seduce him I can, but I have to work on it. And not a day goes past when he doesn't kiss and hold and touch me. Often he will simply fondle my breasts and although it doesn't lead to intercourse I never feel that I am not desired by him.

'As a man he is an interesting mixture; he likes football and having a few beers and he can appear quite gruff and macho. But he is also extremely feminine and gentle, more likely to do the nurturing and caring in our relationship than I am. He so hates the sadness caused by the rigid ways of being a man in which men are unable to express their emotions. He's freed himself from those constraints.

'I don't know what he says about his sex life in front of other men, but he wouldn't feel he has to impress anybody. He's not at all influenced by peer pressure. He would only be concerned about the difference in our levels of desire if he thought I was upset by it, but as long as things are good between us it really doesn't matter.'

'I am training him to please me.'

'Our sex life has got better with time. I am involved in an ongoing process of training him to please me. It used to be more a matter of him getting what he wants, but I also feel that I deserve to get what I want. Although he is very tactile, when it comes to penetration he is more the stereotypical male who goes for orgasm. We're talking about that and how we can refine and work on our lovemaking. Communication is the key to all this.

'I'm interested in working Tantrically *(see Further Reading, Margo Anand)* so that the energy field of my body can weave in with my husband's through the chakras (energy centres). I imagine weaving a figure of eight with his chakras, deepening the connections between us. I can feel this energy field and sometimes I can see it too.

'This is a richer concept of sex than the usual straightforward physical connection. I believe that most partnerships would gain a great deal from doing a little Tantric work. My spiritual life is an equally strong focus for my energies as my relationship. A strong spiritual foundation makes a relationship much easier to handle.'

'I have strong sexual desires outside of our relationship.'

'I find that monogamy is a difficult thing; it is hard not to have desires outside of a relationship. But very few people I know have managed to keep an open relationship going.

'I have strong sexual desires outside of our relationship, but I certainly don't act on them as I know that he wouldn't be unfaithful to me and that if I was unfaithful it would rock our relationship very dramatically. I like to be loyal and I'm not interested in deceit, so the most appropriate thing is not to follow these desires.

'But I do think about sex a lot; quite often it is at the forefront of my mind. I am aware of my desire for both men and women – which is a very different thing from falling in love. Even so, I'd probably be happier in a different culture where it might be possible to have sexual liaisons without causing problems on the home front.

'I don't deny my sexual feelings and I try not repress them. I acknowledge them to myself, I talk about them with friends – and they do dissipate with time so I don't dwell on them.'

'An all-consuming relationship makes it hard to be happy.'

'I don't bring my desires for other people into my relationship with my husband because that would be a kind of dishonesty, an emotional disloyalty. If I fantasize during sex it is about more archetypal figures, god-like images. Fantasy is a kind of energy.

'It's also fair to say that my relationship is only one part of my life, it is not all-consuming. When a relationship is the driving force in your life, it is very hard to be happy.'

'Sex was fantastic at first; now it has changed and gone deeper.'

Richard, 28, has been with his girlfriend Rachel, 26, for nearly three years. They have been living together for half that time. Their sex life – which got off to a frantic start – is now calming down, but her sex drive is higher than his.

Richard:

'As corny as it sounds we've really clicked in a massive way. It's all been pretty amazing and I'm very happy. It took me totally by surprise; I wanted to have some fun and go out with someone – and I just didn't know that it was going to be this good.

'It was only the second time we had met when we spent a lunchtime in a pub talking – it was a real meeting of minds – and then proceeded to drink the afternoon and evening away too. Things moved on very fast from there with the aid of ridiculous amounts of inebriation. There don't seem to be any long courtships any more, at least not for me.

'Sex was fantastic from the very start. It seemed as if we were in bed all the time, at least for the first week. It was pretty frantic. We were already both quite experienced sexually before we met and we felt quite relaxed about everything.

'Things have changed with time and we both talk about the different stages of love. There is that initial period of obsessive passion; then when you become more familiar with each other it goes deeper and changes. Sexually, things level out more.'

'It's usually me who says I don't feel like it…'

'Rachel would be well up for it almost every night, but it's me that's usually tired and not feeling like it. We generally do it about two or three times a week these days, but we have plenty of cuddling and holding as well. There are also some nights when she's too knackered for sex.

'But if we leave it for more than about four or five days, then there is definitely a need for physical release. At that point we either realize what's going on, or we have a row – and then realize it.

'We have a pretty balanced relationship. Rachel is quite concerned not to become like the "mum", and as I was brought up in a feminist household I'm probably more domesticated than she is. We both cook and I'm certainly more concerned with cleanliness, although when it comes to a crisis I probably do over-rely on her.

'Another important side of our relationship is that we are both keen on our careers. We have a shared aim of doing something creative, and so far it is working out very well. We talk about our work a lot, although sometimes I think I don't listen to her enough.

'Sex is good fun so it's a shame not to have more of it, but sometimes I just feel totally knackered. It's partly my job; partly the result of having a few beers and staying up too late. If I smoke cigarettes as well, that totally does me in.'

'I sometimes feel bad about saying no to her.'

'I really like mutual foreplay and massage; I'm totally into it. If there's no sex at the end of it I might feel a bit pissed off! We are both very sensuous people; we enjoy our food a lot too.

I don't worry much about my male identity in not being up for it when she is, although I do sometimes feel quite bad about saying no to her. Generally I will roll over and say I'm sleepy. She grumbles a bit, and then we go to sleep. She's a very physical person and sometimes she will pinch me or tickle me to make me laugh – which releases the tension of the situation. Fortunately, we have a similar sense of humour.'

Rachel:

'We met when we were at university, chatting with a group of friends. I got talking to him and thought he a was nice man – but then didn't see him again until nine months later. We got chatting again and had a really interesting conversation. He had a beard at the time, which was a bit off-putting, but even so I invited him to dinner that night with another friend.'

'Gentle heavy petting marred by alcohol.'

'We had a few glasses of wine and I thought he was really nice, so he ended up staying. We kind of half-heartedly jumped into bed together. We ended up in a sort of gentle heavy petting session marred by lack of co-ordination due to alcohol.

'I woke up the next morning and instead of thinking "oh no, what have I done!", I thought "maybe we could go for a walk together or something". So we drank coffee and played Scrabble and I just didn't want him to leave.

'He went out that night with his parents, but I couldn't wait to see him again. He came round the next day with a bag of cherries and some cheese and we went for a picnic. He had shaved his beard off too! We spent the next fortnight solidly together. It was amazing; that really intense feeling of intoxication. There is no bigger high.

'I had lost my virginity at 19 because I was bored with being the only one who couldn't join in the conversations about sex. But it was miserable and I wondered what all the fuss was about. I'd moved on from there before I met Richard, but I was hardly a multi-orgasmic woman!'

'Too much in love to make love.'

'Richard and I didn't actually make love until three days after we first slept together. We were doing so much and talking so much that we were both shattered. And I think we were both in a state of wonder with each other; I was certainly in wonder of him. So it just didn't happen at first, not until it felt like the right moment. It brought us really, really close.

'And it was one of the first very satisfying sexual experiences of my life. It did feel really special. I've never believed the old idea that women need emotion to enjoy sex whereas men can be purely physical, but this was a coming together of the physical and emotional.

'I've had to educate myself in what my body can do and what feels right. It's been a learning process for me that didn't really start until I was 20 and discovered a women's health book belonging to my mother which described masturbation. But the first time we made love he knew what my body was doing. He was responding to me, feeling my responses, listening to my body.'

'He asked me to tell him my desires.'

'Although sex was brilliant from the beginning with Richard, it has got better with him as we have grown more sensitive to each other. We have learned to love each other's bodies more.

'He also asked me things like – have you had an orgasm? What would you like me to do? That was totally a shock to me because no one had ever asked me those things before.

'I was a bit embarrassed at first because it meant that I had to deal with my own desires and communicate them to him. But it was also very exciting because he was allowing me to be myself. It was terrifying to begin with, but the message was "I welcome your desires".'

'The heart-fluttering died down – but we moved on.'

'I've always been a romantic and I used to have intense infatuations with men. But we always reached a point where the fluttering of my heart died down and I thought "help, I'm not in love any more".

'But Richard was different. There was a solid base underneath and an intellectual connection. My heart-fluttering did die down after about six months and we reached that crisis period – but instead of panicking that it was over we moved on. That was a big turning point for me. It was also after six months that we moved in together, which just felt very natural.

'I realized that what we had was deeper than sexual infatuation. It didn't matter that the desire dies down; it comes back again. I still get that heart-fluttering feeling with Richard sometimes – seeing him after he has been away for a few days, or seeing him across a dinner table when we go out. I look at him being witty and lovely and I think "ooh, gosh! Isn't he wonderful – and he's mine!"'

'Our sex life slows down and then picks up again.'

'We both work full time now and that has slowed our sex life down a bit. One of us goes to bed and falls asleep and that's it. Our sex life reaches these plateaus and then builds up again. We slow down to doing it about two or three times a week – like Saturday night, Sunday morning – and then it picks up again, usually when we find ourselves in unfamiliar situations.

'When you are in your own house it is so easy to get wrapped up in your own thoughts. But if we go away for the weekend, for instance, or if we go out and do things together, it reminds me of how much I love him. I fall in love with him all over again, and then I want to make love to him.

'I have a higher sex drive than he has. Sometimes it's uncomfortable for me; sometimes it's plain frustrating. I do sometimes feel guilty about it. It's difficult if you want something all the time. The truth is that Richard and I are the polar opposites of the myths about women and men. I have wondered if I am abnormal – or if I am just internalizing our culture's disapproval of women's desires.'

'When I want to make love
and he doesn't – then we have a bit of a row.'

'Sometimes I annoy him when I want to make love and he doesn't. I'll prod him in bed and say "come on! wake up!" – and then we have a bit of a row. But it's so absurd, you're rowing because you love someone and want to make love – so we usually end up laughing. Or because I'm quite physical we end up having a pillow fight which defuses some of my frustration.

'When I've calmed down a bit I'll decide to wake him up to make love early the next morning, and then I'll read a book. Or I end up masturbating, but I find that's difficult to accept. It is something I can enjoy, but it's not the same as having sex. I have this deep-rooted feeling – which I am consciously trying to overcome – that I shouldn't be doing it when I am in the same bed as somebody else.

'It's not just about coming. Making love is about being very very close to your partner. It's not just a matter of having an orgasm; it can be about trust, or feeling lonely. Sometimes I am feeling horny, but sometimes I may be feeling insecure. It's all far more loaded than just sexual "passion".

'Sex. Making love. Fucking. They are distinct activities. We only have a handful of words to describe these things, and that is not enough.'

'It's harder for me to say no.'

'The fact that my sex drive is higher than Richard's does affect my perception of him. Sometimes it makes me think that he is a lot more in control of himself, in the sense that he can voice his desire – or his lack of desire. That makes me angry at times, with my self and with him. It seems unfair.

'I have difficulty in saying "no" or "I'm tired" to him. It makes me think – "God, he's so able to say what he's thinking and feeling, while I don't feel able to do that". A lot of my frustration is that I find it difficult to be so assertive'.

'As far as domestic stuff is concerned, I'm a bit crap. I cook, he cleans, it balances out. I do believe in being faithful. We don't have an open relationship; I've got no plans to go off with anyone else and I hope Richard hasn't. But I wouldn't be rabid about it. If it did happen I'd like to think that we could work it out.'

'We have huge rows – and it's alright.'

'We row a lot about everything, from big issues like politics to "why didn't you buy any cheese today?"! I have never rowed with anyone like this before. Huge, screaming rows – and then it's alright again. I've learned that one argument doesn't mean the end of the relationship and that is incredibly important to me.

'Only a month before I met Richard I was crying to my mother about how so many men just seemed to be wankers. But then I met him and it was so right. We are from very similar backgrounds; we read the same books; we talk about the same things. He is definitely Mr Right as far as I'm concerned and I would like us to get married and have children eventually. I'm happy being partners for the time being, but it would be good to have a big celebration of our commitment to each other.'

Surviving the Bad Patch – and Rediscovering Passion

Marcus and Anne have been married for 17 years. About seven years into their relationship they struck such stormy waters that they stopped sleeping together and came close to splitting up. Yet today their relationship is on an even keel once more, and they say their sex life is better than ever.

Marcus:

'Friends thought we were "the perfect couple"…'

'We met on a beach in Spain and fell in love when we were in our early 20s. It was all very romantic, and to our friends and colleagues we were "the perfect couple".

'After that, and until we had children, we were very busy growing together and building a home. We are at our best when we are doing things together and we seemed to have no problems. Sex was a regular thing and an important form of communication. We had more lust in those days – I suppose we used to make love about three or four times a week.

'At the beginning of our relationship, I knew that Anne had been in a long-term relationship before we met and that made me feel very insecure. Would I be as good as her previous lover? My first serious love affair was with a woman who hardly allowed any physical contact – although she had a lover before me – for a period of four years. The pain of that situation for me was intense, and I still return to it in my dreams.

'But the physical side of my relationship with Anne was wonderful. Although I had about 13 or 14 different lovers before I met Anne, I still regard her as the most attractive woman I've ever seen or touched. I've not wanted to touch anyone else since we got married 17 years ago. She is also my best friend.'

'I was stressed, depressed – and we didn't make love for months.'

'Then – after about seven years – I got a new job and we moved house. We had two young children at the time and Anne had become very insular, at home with the children all day, whilst I wasn't very good at being selfless with them.

'I was coming home feeling very stressed and depressed, with a lot of work still to do. All I wanted was a cuddle, but that was the last thing I'd get. I thought at the time it was the worst move we had ever made because everything seemed to go wrong after that. It was horrendous.

'When it went wrong I couldn't understand what was happening. There was an enormous emotional impact on our relationship and a period of about six months when we didn't make love at all. I felt terribly rejected.

'It was so painful and so lonely that I ended up one day in a supermarket car park, weeping my eyes out. I thought I had made the worst move of my life. At times we had to call friends over to talk to us, because I was just sobbing at the kitchen table. I remember hitting the floor so hard that my fist has never been the same since.

'We had two years of that. It was chiefly a difficulty in communicating with each other. We returned again and again to the same issues – until I started listening and Anne started to be able to say what she wanted to say. The fact that she went back into education in the meantime made all the difference.'

'Emotionally, we had won the Lottery.'

'After she went out and got her degree I felt as if – emotionally – we had won the Lottery. With her new self-belief and self-confidence our ability to communicate was so much better. Anne used to jokingly chant "2:1" at me – because she got a top second degree, whereas I got a 2:2. But I rejoiced in her achievement.

'One of the things we did was to make Friday nights absolutely sacrosanct. We very rarely went out, even if we were invited to dinner. We needed to have time together at home. We would feed the kids early, get them off to bed and sit down to watch *Gardeners' World* (we both love gardening) on the television. After that we would have something nice to eat – just for us – and a good bottle of wine. And we would talk.

'On our Friday evenings we frequently ended up making love too. It would happen downstairs rather than in the bedroom, which is a different kind of lovemaking.

'These days there is a bit of a problem with Friday nights which is that our children are teenagers, so they don't go to bed early any more. I'm concerned that – given how unrelaxed Anne is about sex when we have visitors in the house – she is going to find their continual presence a problem. And if she wants to dress in something sexy they are going to ask – why are you wearing that Mum? Or more to the point, why are you not wearing that?

'But that is what happens to sex in a long-term relationship. We are continually making adjustments, so we have to be inventive. If our physical relationship didn't have to negotiate those changes it would probably come to an end through boredom. But because we continually make these positive adjustments, it leads to variations in our lovemaking. Life imposes change which keeps things alive between us.'

'Sometimes we make love without preamble – at other times we are more lusty and rude!'

'We haven't had a comparable period of sexual inactivity since those difficult two years, except for shorter spells when we go on holiday or we have other people staying in the house. At those times Anne can't relax enough to enjoy making love.

'Sometimes we make love with hardly any preamble. At other times we are more lusty and premeditated and rude! I usually initiate lovemaking – I would say 99 per cent of the time. I've often wondered what would happen if I didn't initiate it but I have no sense that she is fulfilling a dutiful role; her response is a positive one. If I felt she was making love out of a sense of duty I'd hate that. Routine, duty and expectations: those are the real passion killers.

'But I'm not unhappy with the way we function. In the rest of our relationship we have developed different roles – when it comes to cooking and decorating and looking after the children. It's the same when it comes to making love.'

'Making love has become a celebration of our relationship.'
'Our physical relationship at its best is a real celebration of who we are with each other. This is a very different thing from being young and "needing a fuck" – which is really just a release of sexual tension. You might just as well spend 20 or 30 quid to see a prostitute.

'At the beginning of a relationship it is a matter of finding out about the other person, about giving and taking from each other. But you don't have that deep down feeling of knowing that your relationship really works. That comes with time and knowing what makes the relationship tick.

'These days I am no longer thinking – where should I put my hand, what should I do next? We have got to the stage where we can forget about performance. Lovemaking has become less about technique; it is now more emotional and intuitive. It's about trust.

'Now that we are mature, even the sensations of making love feel different, although we are going through the same basic motions. There is a closer quality. It takes many years of making love to get this sense of absolute confidence. It's about knowing someone very intimately. We are closer now than we have ever been – and we just know more.

'When our sexual relationship works well, it's about the whole deal, every aspect of our life together. In our life now there is an equality and a compatibility. We're good in differ-ent – but complementary – areas.

'I feel we've achieved so much together, discovered so much, that our life is almost like a book, the stuff of fantasy. I don't know what the future holds, but it must be interesting.

I have a belief that things will always get better. I want to go travelling with Anne. I want to make love to her somewhere hot and exotic.'

Anne:
'I had to choose between him and the children.'

'At the time when we were going through our difficulties, Marcus was very angry and frustrated. He would bring work home, shout at the kids, feel unhappy – and then want a cuddle from me. The kids would be crying because of all the anger and verbal abuse and I felt I had to protect them. I had to choose between him and the children, and I chose to stand by the children.

'I remember feeling very cold towards him in bed at that time. I didn't even want him to touch me. We even slept in separate rooms. It was an extremely hurtful time. I remember not liking him and not loving him. We very nearly separated.

'It was like a "seven-year itch" in that I needed something more for myself. It might have been a course or it might have been another man. I had to realize what I needed – and it was a university course. We had a very close friend at that time who used to come round to have coffee with me and talk. I felt closer to him than to Marcus. I used to feel happy in his company. There could have been a physical relationship between us – but there wasn't.

'Before that time my relationship with Marcus had never got to the point where we needed to talk about difficult emotions. I found it very hard to talk. I was useless at putting my feelings into words while Marcus was always interrupting what I was trying to say, jumping impatiently on every phrase.'

'I had to learn to talk about my feelings.'

'My family doesn't talk about feelings – at least not negative ones. My mother once said to Marcus – don't talk about emotions please, it's bad manners! So I had to learn to talk about my negative feelings.

'How did we get back with each other? It was various things. I went back to university which gave me a different focus. I had a new passion, new excitement. I needed to feel I was achieving something. At home with the children I was becoming bored, lethargic and deflated. At the end of each day I had nothing to say.

'After I went to university I was happier in myself – and able to share it with Marcus. From there our relationship became physical again.

'I went to see a relationship counsellor, without telling Marcus. I needed someone to listen to me. We also had our friend who came round to see us and who helped us to communicate; we needed that.

'Our Friday evenings together helped too. We would have a bottle of wine together and I would go upstairs and dress in something sexy – and come down again. That's becoming difficult now that our children are older. After 10 o'clock, if they're still around, we start the second bottle of wine – and after that I just want to fall asleep!

'But they do go out sometimes, to sleepovers and to friends' houses. I've thought of making an arrangement with a friend who has kids the same age; we could swap them on alternate weekends!

'Sometimes I'm hoping the kids are going to go out so that we can have some time together, but then they don't. We have to make adjustments all the time. But that's one of the good things about sex in a long-term relationship: it's not predictable. The thing that will turn me on one time won't work another time. It's all about psychology and mood.'

'No sex makes him grumpy – which makes me stubborn…'

'If Marcus and I haven't made love for three or four days I notice that he changes as a person. He becomes less tolerant. It's almost a hormonal thing; he seems to get angry if we haven't made love, and then he relaxes after we have.

'I do feel there are times, when we have friends staying here or when I'm tired, that he gets angry and I get stubborn. I realize it's because we haven't made love for a while, but I'm not going to do it unless I want to. I think, why should I? I'm a person; I'm me, I don't have to do this just because he's grumpy.

'Sometimes when we've cooled down with each other sexually, the tension builds up into a spiral. For me it helps to nip the situation in the bud if we dress up and go out with friends. Then I can see Marcus from a different perspective. I quite fancy him when I see him across a dinner table! We do warm to each other when we go out.'

'I don't feel I will go berserk without sex.'

'In the long term, that period of difficulty did our relationship a power of good. When you are at home with two young children you feel you have no contact with the rest of the world. By going to university I got my life back. It changed me as a person, improved my self-image no end – and I was so excited by my studies that I wanted to share it all with Marcus – who works in the same field. We had such conversations!

'Nowadays we have got a good balance, but I think Marcus needs the physical side of our relationship more than I do. I never feel that if I don't have sex I will go berserk, whereas he usually initiates sex.

'We still fancy each other, but it's deeper than in the early days. It involves everything we've been through and shared – including my father's death, Marcus going through a serious illness and worries about losing our home.'

'I enjoy giving pleasure more slowly, more deliberately.'

'And now we each know exactly what turns the other on. Our physical relationship is more fulfilling. At the beginning of a relationship you don't bother with any "extras" or props or sexy clothes; you just get on with it in a hurry! Sometimes we do make love quickly, but usually it's a longer process. As I've got older I have enjoyed being able to give pleasure more slowly and deliberately.

'I feel that our relationship is equal. We both cook and share jobs in the house. He does his own ironing; we both work. It means that we don't have any build-up of resentment. We also do a lot together in the house. We always work together, so that if I'm doing wallpapering, Marcus will be sanding the windows. If he is in the kitchen cooking, I will chop the vegetables and we will have a glass of wine together and talk.

'At the beginning of our relationship the sexual side was brilliant, and it's brilliant now, but there are more things we do now, more variety. If Marcus died and I had a new relationship it would be totally different. This relationship is unique. It changes and evolves and grows as we do.'

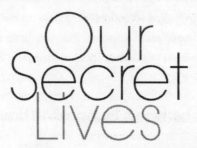

CHAPTER 2

Our Secret Lives

One of the Last Taboos

When did you last talk openly about your sex life – apart from jokey allusions to the lack of it? If you are in a long-term relationship, chances are you just don't discuss the matter and that you have no idea what anyone else is up to either.

'Sex in long-term relationships really is one of the last taboos,' says Denise Knowles of UK counselling organization Relate. 'No matter whether the sex is good or bad, as people get older, the topic gets eased out of the conversation.'

Why? First, there is embarrassment. We might think we are a broad-minded, sexually liberated society, yet the reality is that we simply do not talk about such things after we have 'settled down'.

Secondly, there is loyalty. It's all very well confiding about Great Sex I Have Had when you are (or were) young and fancy free, but once you are in an established couple there is your partner to consider.

How is he going to feel if you have spilled the beans about that fantastic (or perhaps completely hopeless) night you spent at a hotel while your mum looked after the kids? How can she be comfortable at your next dinner party knowing that you have told the person beside you about her preference for cunnilingus?

'It's his birthday; I suppose I'll have to…'

And then there are your friends to consider. You may be having a fantastic time in bed with your partner of many years, yet your best friend has hinted to you that her sex life with her husband has completely ground to a halt. Says Karen:

I'd love to be able to talk to my two best friends about my sex life, but how can I? One of them is getting divorced at the moment and says she's so desperate she'd bonk anything in trousers. Meanwhile my other friend is saying things like – it's his birthday so I'll suppose I'll have to!

If I were to tell them what a good time we are having, they would only feel worse. They might even think I was bragging.

And then there's the haunting suspicion that our friends may be having a much better time in bed than we are. 'Twice a week!' you confide, glowing with pride. 'Poor old you!' they sigh, 'only twice a week!'

It is a can of worms and, not surprisingly, most couples do keep quiet about the details of their sex lives.

The Downside of Discretion

Unfortunately, our widespread reticence about sex in long relationships has several negative consequences. As Julia Cole of Relate puts it, we don't know the etiquette of sex because we don't know what anyone else is doing:

If someone was cooking for you, you could say – I like my egg done for four-and-a-half minutes please! But we have no comparable way of talking about our sexual preferences.

Our silence about sex hampers our relationships because of:

- FALSE ASSUMPTIONS. It fosters the false assumption that only young people – and/or the newly in love – have good sex. The truth is that people who have been together for a long time often have plenty of sex which is more inventive, stimulating and deeply satisfying than anything they experienced in their early days.
- ISOLATION. When we go through 'bad patches' we may fear that it's all over. Yet if we can hang on in there, realizing that every long relationship has its times of ebb and flow, we may have years of pleasure ahead together.
- INHIBITIONS. When sex is a taboo subject, how can we talk to our partners about what we enjoy – or what we dislike?
- ANXIETY ABOUT BEING 'NORMAL'. We may worry about whether we are 'normal'? Should we be trying harder? Could things be better? Or should we be hanging up our suspender belts and 'growing old gracefully'?

- NOT FACING PROBLEMS. Sexual problems can be an early indicator of relationship problems. If you can't talk about them, it's hard to seek help – and so harder to keep your relationship on the road.

The Big Ban on sex talk can start almost immediately in a relationship, intensifying to solid silence as the years go by. And by the time you've clocked up 10, 20 – or more – years, it's a hard habit to break.

As a result, most of us have no idea how it really is for other couples. All we know is what tabloid newspapers and women's magazines tell us – that on average, other people are doing it twice a week. That's enough to make us feel bad if we aren't; smug if we are. But fascinating as it is to look at the figures – usually the only hint we ever get about what our fellow humans are up to in bed – bald statistics tell us nothing about the quality or intensity of that sex, nothing about the amount of love and affection in those relationships.

At Your Age!

Much of the Big Ban on sex talk is to do with age. Says Denise Knowles:

There is a general perception that now you've had your children and so on, sex just doesn't happen. There is a widespread notion that we should not be enjoying sex in the long term. But a lot of my girlfriends are in their 40s and 50s and when the subject does come up they start giggling, almost like teenaged girls, as if to say – at my age I shouldn't be thinking like this!

Because we have grown up with these stereotypes, if we find we are having a good sex life in our middle years we can't be comfortable. Therefore we perpetuate the stereotypes, even when they do not fit with our experience.

Kate, a mother of two who has been married for 12 years, just doesn't accept the stereotype:

People still make the same old assumption that women who have been in a relationship for a long time just don't want sex any more. It makes me so cross! My sex life is absolutely great!

When I was at university I read *The Hite Report*. I had been completely ignorant and found it incredibly helpful and informative. That's why I'm prepared to talk about my sex life for this book. I've got one woman friend I would discuss sex with, but then only in general terms, never the details. I think it's a shame we don't discuss these things more openly.

Notches on the Bedpost

For what it's worth:

- Most sexually active people in Britain do it two or three times a week. Four per cent of the population claim to do it every day.

- Most lusty are people in the southwest of England, who claim to do it on average 85 times a year. Least lusty are the natives of central-southern Britain, who clock up around 68 times a year per head.
  (Source: Durex Report, 1994)

- Four out of ten single women (aged 16 to 49) are celibate.
  (Source: General Household Survey, 1995)

Myth No. 1: 'Sex Stops at a Certain Age'

There are two big myths about youth and age which directly affect the way we think about our sex lives. The first is that sex is not for older people.

For many in our mothers' generation (when sex was a man's 'right'), 'the change' meant the end of sex – and what a relief! According to psychosexual counsellor Jane Hawksley of Relate:

Historically, menopause was a time to give up on sex. But things have changed, there is no question about it, since the advent of the Pill in the 1960s. The children of the '60s are now hitting middle age, and they still adhere to the culture of being forever young.

This has blazed a trail, but in addition we now have HRT, so that the extreme symptoms of the menopause – like loss of libido and a dry vagina – no longer have to have a significant impact. Today, women are encouraged to be sexually active for longer and sex in old age is considered important.

Now that HRT is available, you are no longer finished in middle age.

These days the notion of the sexy older woman is in vogue (especially if she appears topless in a television drama). But only if she looks much the same as a sexy young woman – slim, no sagging, no stretch marks. For being 'old' and having sex is still taboo, and our mothers' voices still echo in our minds, telling us it's time to hang up the negligee and invest in separate beds.

Myth No. 2: 'Sex is Good When You Are Young'

The second big myth, flipside of the first, is that Sex is Always Wonderful When You Are Young. But just cast your mind back to your early sexual experiences, or ask your friends – and it's a different story.

Sue is 39:

I made a conscious effort to get rid of my virginity when I was about 16. It was disastrous. You know what they say about pushing marshmallows into letterboxes? Well, that's what it was like. It really upset me and put me off sex for an entire year.

Then I fell in love with an older man and had sex with him. But I didn't even know the word 'orgasm', let alone have any experience of it. I was quite innocent, very repressed and embarrassed about sex. It wasn't a matter of having 'moral' ideas about sex; I was just desperately self-conscious. I was very impressed by a girlfriend of mine who said her boyfriend knew how to make her come without having penetrative sex at all!

When I first got together with my husband I was utterly passive. I just lay there and did very little. We had lots of caressing and cuddling, but definitely no oral sex – not for years. We were so serious in bed. We never talked during sex, or laughed. I realized later that he was also doubting his sexuality. He was politically aware and concerned about male domination; it was a time when women were asking if penetrative sex was a good idea at all!

In short, we weren't tremendously lustful. In fact I didn't experience real lust for a long time.

Fiona is 35:

My early sexual experiences were pretty awful. Being groped by spotty boys with dirt under their fingernails at school dances. Going home with purple love bites on my neck after parties. Not knowing what bits of him to touch, or to let him touch.

I lost my virginity at 17 and it was hilarious. I lay on my back with my legs spread, but he couldn't penetrate me – until we discovered that I needed to bend my knees a bit!

Several boyfriends later and well into university I still hadn't had an orgasm. Then when I really fell for someone and was desperately keen for it all to work, I was so tense that he couldn't penetrate me at all. Disaster!

Not until many years later when I was well into a lasting relationship was there enough love and trust for me to really enjoy myself.

Suzanne is in her 50s:

When I was 19 I had an affair with an actor who was twice my age. It was safe territory; I knew he wasn't in love with me, and I wasn't in love with him either, but we enjoyed each other.

I told him that I was a virgin, but if he was prepared to hang on for a couple of weeks then he could make love to me. I found a doctor who gave me a prescription for the Pill. It was 1965 and it cost half a guinea for a private consultation.

I broke my own hymen with a hairbrush handle before we went to bed together. I wanted to do it myself because I needed to feel in control of what was going on.

It was a great relief to have lost my virginity without any great emotional upheaval. It was all very well planned and deliberate. Technically I was proficient in sex – but it was many years before I experienced real passion.

The Great Sexual Unlocking

Fortunately, for most women these dodgy or even disastrous beginnings are followed by a time when things get dramatically better. Many of us look back on this time with great nostalgia, as our Golden Age of Sex, the times when we never did it so good.

Sue again:

I went straight into an affair with a lecturer when I was at university. He was 10 years older than me and that was the unlocking of my sexuality. I can remember lying in bed and thinking 'this is frightening – to feel this strongly'. Sex was all. We were completely obsessive and I was burned up totally. It was the first time I had ever experienced that. I was glowing and hot for it!

Fiona again:

Then in my early 20s I met a much older, married man who completely swept me off my feet. For about a year I was completely obsessed by him and our sex life was extraordinary. We couldn't keep our hands off each other, even in public, and when we did get a whole night together we would make love three or four times – and always in the morning as well. When we couldn't spend a night together we would do it anywhere that we could find: once in the back of a taxi, once in a graveyard! I just had to think of him and I would be close to orgasm.

Liz is 37, **married with three children:**

I was a very horny person before I had children. Sex was very much a part of my energy. It was my power when I walked into a room and saw how men looked at me. I felt – right, I can get whatever I want.

Ellie is 42:

I was really wild when I was about 18, before I met up with my husband. If I met a bloke I liked, I took him home and shagged him. It was simply an extension of liking someone.

Caroline is 32:

When we were first married, if it got to the end of the week and we hadn't made love I would get really upset. When we were courting we sometimes used to do it three or four times in an afternoon – and then a couple of times after supper and again in the morning. We would think nothing of it.

Nicky is 34:

I used to do it anywhere and everywhere, up trees, in pick-up trucks, on the kitchen table, you name it…It was always much nicer than being in bed.

Garden of Eden

Remember the days when we answered to no one? No to the bosses. No to the phone. No to the doorbell. No to the clock. Read to each other. Fed each other. Dressed and undressed each other. Adam and Eveing 'til Kingdom come.

From *LOVEBITES*, a play by Tom Clark.

Lost Lust?

Many of us look back on those days and think 'what happened?' For with the Great Sexual Unlocking comes freedom. But freedom brings choices, such as – will I marry him, or won't I? Is this a long-term commitment, and if so, are we going to have children together?

Yet commitment and children are often incompatible with great sex. According to researcher Shere Hite, people tend not to settle with or marry the one who gave them the best sex ever. Traditionally, men have divided women into two separate camps: lovers and wives, or 'bad' girls and 'good'. In the simplest terms, the 'bad' ones are good for sex, but the 'good' ones are those who end up with the wedding ring.

Women, too, make the same kinds of choices, consciously or otherwise, about who will make a good father and a provider. 'I knew he wanted children' we say, or 'I knew I could rely on him'.

Unromantic and calculating – or plain common sense? Throughout history, most people the world over have married on this basis. In spite of our ideals of free and romantic love, it seems we are not so different.

Says Barbara:

I've been wanting babies since I was 16, although I didn't have my first until I was 33. It was a condition of getting married for me. I was pregnant on my wedding day.

According to Emily:

I was 19 when we got married and I always assumed that we would have children. I don't think I would have been with him if he wasn't fond of children. I've always known that it was the main thing I wanted in life.

For many of us, then, our choice of life partner is not based on rampant desire in the first place. Which makes it a bit unfair to compare our long-term lover with one we may have known in our fondly remembered Golden Age.

Even if we do settle with or marry the sexual love of our lives, we are likely to find that 'first lust' doesn't last.

Liz has been married for 10 years:

Now with three children under the age of eight, I'm completely different. I find it hard not to have that power now, the power of sexual energy. Instead of wanting to have wild sex all the time, it's 'Poor bloke, it's been two weeks, I'd better do it!' We still have our raunchy phases, but he's almost like my brother now. We've got such a close friendship that we've lost that sexual mystery of the stranger.

Fiona has been with her partner for 16 years:

After the first year or two, the urgency wore off. We still enjoyed it, but I was no longer bent double with desire if I hadn't seen him for a day or two. The notion of going to bed to go to sleep crept into our relationship. Our courtship phase, it seemed, was over.

The Problem with Passion

Many of us look back with regret to those days of frantic sex, as if they were the pinnacle of our love lives. We mourn for a time when arousal seemed to be instant and orgasm was something to be held in check, rather than worked for. But what would life be like if we kept up that kind of sexual pace, great bags under our eyes and thinking of nothing but the next bunk up?

Says Jane Hawksley of Relate:

The excitement and spontaneity of the courtship phase is a very important underpinning to a relationship, but you can't sustain that. We would all be worn out! Yet people long for it to return. They complain that sex in a long-term relationship is no longer exciting, no longer spontaneous. But people's ideas of sex are completely unrealistic.

The problem with passion is that it is not always compatible with earning a living and enjoying domestic peace, stability and harmony, not to mention sleep. In other words, passion is something that you can quite easily do without in the long struggle to make a home and bring up children.

Yet many of us still do cling, quite unreasonably, to the idea that we should or could be able to get back to that stage of our relationship.

Which is not to say that spontaneity and lust do not resurface in long relationships, or that sex becomes dull and dutiful for the rest of our lives. The truth is that after the intense bonding of the courtship phase, we embark upon a long journey which can include bad times and good times.

We may meet many obstacles to intimacy. Maintaining a relationship can at times be very hard work, and we may – for a time at least – simply give up on sex with our partners. But for countless women and their men, the long-term rewards of a sustained sexual relationship are rich, varied and well worth waiting for.

As Kate puts it:

Although the quantity of our sexual encounters has diminished, the quality has certainly increased. When we do it now, we do it good!

The following chapters chart some of the ups and downs of this journey, offering some markers and buoys from other couples who are travelling the same choppy seas.

CHAPTER 3

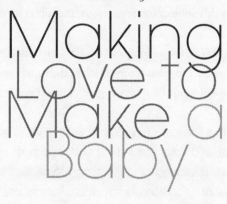

Making Love to Make a Baby

Of all the life events which can ambush your sex life leaving it in tatters, having a baby is often the most significant. This chapter looks at how parenthood can change your sex life. It may get better. It may get worse. Whatever happens, after babies it will never be the same again.

An Alien Experience?

Picture this. An alien lands in a newsagent anywhere in the western world. Shelf after shelf of magazines and newspapers shout 'SEX!' in big letters. (Please note that this book shouts it in small letters.)

'Sex for fun!' 'Sex for orgasms!' 'Sex for the sake of it!'

But what about reproduction, wonders the alien? How ever do they do *that*? Or is this subject too mysterious, too taboo for earthlings to mention?

Often, it seems, we no longer make the link between having sex and having babies. But what we overlook at the same time is that trying to make a baby can be a very highly charged erotic experience:

If I'm ovulating, I'm just raring to go! When I want to conceive I do have a wild time sexually. The freedom to conceive is tremendously liberating and exciting. I think that contraception is a great passion killer. As soon as I stopped the Pill I had a stronger sexual appetite.

I was on the Pill for a long time – having tried everything else – and then I gave up the whole lot. Suddenly, physically and psychologically, I felt a wonderful release. Is it because you are doing it for the first time to try to make a baby? Or is it because you are being given permission to do it? These days I can feel the 'ping' in mid-cycle as I ovulate – and I'm ready!

We were moving house and the condoms had already gone into the packing cases inside the bedside cabinet. We started making love on top of the packing cases. But I was well aware of my hormonal cycle, and knowing that I was in the fertile period I said 'We really shouldn't be doing this!' He said – just 30 seconds prior to conception – 'Why not?', and mentioned friends of ours who had just had a baby. I thought – 'Great! Off we go!' It was wonderful. I just knew we would conceive, and we did.

Pregnancy Can Be a Big Turn-on

A woman's body changes dramatically with pregnancy, and as those breasts and bellies swell, some women – and their men – find pregnancy a major turn-on:

I loved sex during pregnancy; you can be very engorged 'down there' because of the pressure of the baby on your pelvis. Before getting pregnant I had been a 'twice daily' woman, and during pregnancy those feelings came back. It was wonderful!

I loved the bodily changes of pregnancy. Sex was terrific and we bonked frantically right up to the end. I was really randy, panting for it! Being thin wasn't a worry any more; all the anxieties dropped away. I felt I looked beautiful – we both did – and sexually we had a very good time.

Some couples are delighted to find that they are equally keen to carry on having sex as soon as physically possible after the birth. A National Childbirth Trust (NCT) survey (1995) of 1,000 mothers in the UK found that 16 per cent of women felt their sex life was better after childbirth. For having a baby is a profound experience which can make women feel confident, strong and truly womanly as never before:

My son was born by elective caesarean because I have a funny-shaped pelvis. But as soon as I got home we looked at each other and thought – never mind the six-week check, we can't wait! It was lovely having sex again without the bump in the way. I used to leak milk when I came, but he loved that. He called it our DIY bed Jacuzzi.

We had carried on having sex right up until the day of the birth; in fact we were hard at it for days because the baby was overdue and we had been told that sex could trigger off contractions. But I had no idea what to expect after the baby. I had a small tear and stitches in my perineum, but to my surprise, breastfeeding made me feel incredibly sexual. I was just dying to have sex again – which we did within a couple of weeks. Of course, we were both thinking about the birth as he penetrated me, but he just said, 'The last person to be here was our baby.' Just that acknowledgement made it all okay.

Tiredness, Stitches and the Infant Sex Police

For others – particularly women who already have young children – the tiredness and nausea of pregnancy is overwhelming, and sex is the last thing on their minds. Indeed the whole business of new parenthood brings profound changes to any relationship.

At one level, your self-image as a lover is likely to have been changed by the process of childbirth. As our alien in the newsagent noticed, we tend to regard certain parts of a woman – especially her vagina and breasts – to be exclusively for sex. These are the bits which men are supposed to lust after. These are the bits which it is rude – but highly erotic – to reveal.

Then, suddenly, childbirth takes over these bits and in the process they can get quite a battering. It's difficult for couples to regard them in quite the same light for a while. And if the birth has been a difficult one, the consequences for your sex life can last for some time:

I'm a midwife and I talk to many women who have had diffi-cult deliveries, and their sex life is affected for a long time afterwards. Even a normal birth can leave feelings that take a lot of exorcizing.

I can't forget those high forceps and that awful feeling of being invaded. When we have sex it brings back memories of the pain.

After a painful birth, just having something in the vagina can feel as if you are reliving a trauma. It's awful.

Even when the birth is a 'normal' one, weeks of postnatal bleeding, breastfeeding and broken nights can add up to a period of celibacy for many new parents. Sex often takes a nose dive for months, or even years:

The problem started after our first baby was born. We shared a bed with him, and that was it. And anyway, I didn't feel remotely attractive what with milk pads in my bra, other pads in my knickers. My self-image was abysmal. But you have to watch out because you can just get out of the habit. That time of celibacy expanded into two months, then three, four, five! And still we hadn't done it! It became a problem.

We've had periods of abstinence of about six months, all children related, but he never pressurized me. It wasn't just the postnatal period; I had other gynaecological problems, plus extreme tiredness. The months just went by.

He never showed any frustration or impatience, but I felt he was frightened to approach me because he didn't know how I would react.

An NCT (1995) survey of mothers with young children found that, for half of the couples, having a baby made their sex life worse, mostly because of:

- tiredness
- lack of privacy
- lack of libido
- pain from stitches and/or tears.

Utter exhaustion, said mothers, made sleep a more attractive option than sex. One mother characterized her experience like this:

Inappropriate self-image; tiredness; opportunities at the wrong time of the day; vaginal dryness; thrush; infant sex police.

Of course there are good biological reasons for women to go off sex for some time after having babies. Nature wants us to finish breastfeeding one baby before we conceive another, and so fully breastfeeding suppresses ovulation, making conception less likely (but *not* impossible).

When women are breastfeeding they also produce exceptionally high levels of the hormone prolactin which – some researchers believe – reduces sex drive. This could add to the many reasons why new mothers are less likely to initiate sex – yet once sexually aroused, they can enjoy it as much as ever before.

According to psychosexual therapist Jane Hawksley of Relate:

It's not abnormal for couples to go without sex for two years after a baby – although they should start to do something about it by the time the baby is into a routine of better sleeping and less breastfeeding at about six months old. Until then, couples may just have to accept a period of celibacy as one of the realities of new parenthood.

Sex After Motherhood

- Wait until you genuinely feel ready – regardless of the six-week check, which is supposed to be when your stitches are healed, not the date after which you should be 'doing it'.
- If you notice any deep sighs from the other side of the bed, talk it over. Communication is all important.
- Choose your time carefully to discuss things: the middle of the night when the baby is screaming, or during an argument about your relationship is *not* the time to raise the subject. Instead, go out for a drink or a meal – and then start to talk.

- Forget penetration for a while; there are lots of other ways to give each other pleasure and this is a good time to try them out.
- Start slowly and start sensuously. New mothers need TLC as never before. Try lots of gentle touching and massage before you get down to anything more challenging.
- The hormones produced during breastfeeding can also interfere with vaginal lubrication, causing uncomfortable vaginal dryness. Various new vaginal lubricants may help (*see Helpful Organizations in Resources*).
- Women who have had traumatic births may benefit from counselling, together with their partners, to help them come to terms with their experience. Your GP should be able to refer you.

Making Love to Mummy, Making Love to Daddy

There may be another, deeper reason why many people just don't feel like sex after becoming parents – at least not the wild, spontaneous kind of sex we were used to in bygone days. It is that deep in our hearts and minds, we have long since learned that mummies and daddies are not supposed to be sexy:

Apart from all that awful business of the baby hanging on to one breast while the baby's father hangs on to the other – while you just want shot of them both! – the most difficult thing I found about sex after babies was the whole business of becoming 'Mother'. Suddenly, my whole identity had changed. I could no longer see myself as primarily his Lover. Mother loomed larger than Lover, and there is nothing at all sexy about Mother. In fact, Mother and Lover are totally incompatible.

Of course the incest taboos which stop us from thinking of our parents as in any way sexual are very useful, but unfortunately they can also get in the way of sex when *we* become parents.

Think back to your childhood. When you found out about the facts of life (the true story that is), chances are you had to struggle to get your head around the idea that your own mum and dad did that too! Surely they did something different? Or – small consolation – they only did it two or three times to beget you and your siblings!

Julia Cole of Relate has an interesting theory about the long-standing rumour surrounding the Queen – 'mother' of Great Britain – and her husband Prince Philip:

For many years there has been talk that their children were born by some kind of artificial insemination. It strikes me that this has become a kind of modern myth – because people just can't face the idea that our Queen, who is a mother figure, has sex. People have a need to think that 'they must have done it differently', which is why this story has persisted.

Couples talk to me in sex therapy about not being able to believe that their parents had sex. There is an embargo on the whole idea of sex with your father or your mother, which can become mixed up with your own sexual relationship when you become a parent.

Julia Cole has also found from her experience as a psychosexual counsellor for Relate that having children can bring back painful memories from our own childhoods – with implications for our sex lives:

Women might bury memories of abuse to enable them to get on with life and build up a reasonable relationship. But then when their daughters reach the age they were when they were abused, it all comes flooding back.

Or, women could be recalling another traumatic experience, such as bereavement, the arrival of a sibling or bullying, which happened at an age which their children have now reached.

One woman told me that she had been teased about being fat when she was young. The other girls called her names, attacking her chest and her body shape. When her daughter reached the same sort of age, her unresolved emotions about her own childhood were stirred up again, triggering depression.

Getting Sex Started – Hot Tips for New Dads

That new fathers can have a rough time ahead, emotionally and sexually, often gets forgotten in the excitement and turmoil of birth. Yet there are many things men can do to make things better – or worse – on the home front. Here are a few do's and don'ts:

Passion Thrillers

1) Take her out somewhere pleasant and relaxing.
2) When you have had time to talk a bit, catching up on each other's lives, choose your moment carefully to raise the subject.
3) Speaking calmly, say something like 'I am really missing making love to you. How do you feel about it?'
4) Accept the reply she gives you – which might be something like 'I just don't feel like it at the moment.'
5) Ask her if there is anything she would enjoy – and when you get home, try it. Chances are you that you are well on the road to intimacy once more.

Passion Killers

1) Wait until one in the morning when the baby has just dropped off to sleep and so has your partner.
2) Prod her in the back, grab her breast.
3) Sound really desperate when you say your partner's name, putting maximum pressure on her.
4) When she responds with less than total enthusiasm, accuse her of having lost all interest in sex.
5) Roll over in a huff.

Breast Goes West

The extraordinary aversion to breastfeeding in western society is another sign of the sex and mother taboo. In the west (in contrast to the developing world), breasts have become *the* symbol of sex. Of course breasts are sexy – they are an important erogenous zone – but so are other bits of the body.

The reality is that breasts are not just for sex; they are also for feeding babies. Once women are lactating they can leak – even spurt – milk during sex. And it is here, where sex meets motherhood, that men can get horribly uncomfortable.

If men touch their partner's breasts during sex, are they somehow on the baby's 'territory'? Worse still, when the baby sucks at their woman's breast, is this 'sexual'? And another forbidden thought can creep in to spoil your sex life. Is he thinking 'mother' as he caresses your breasts?

Oh, it is all too much! Better just to roll over and go to sleep! But it doesn't have to be that way: some couples do manage to meet the issue head on, so to speak:

We used to have sex when the baby was on my breast. It's odd how the man's head seems so obscenely big on your breast after the tiny head of a baby. In the middle of everything we had to stop and burp the baby. That little head would be bouncing against my breast while I was trying to come. It was hard being a harlot for him and being a mother for the baby at the same time, but I managed it. It's better than leaving the kids crying because you want to come.

Another problem which new parents face is Baby's Intuition. How is it that babies always know when you are – at last – starting to get it together? Is it because they don't want you to make a rival baby? Or are they just natural killjoys?

It never failed to happen. For the first year of our baby's life, he would wake up just at the crucial moment. Not in the early stages when you wouldn't have minded too much, but right at the point of no return when to stop leaves you incredibly frustrated. It nearly drove us round the bend!

Fortunately, some babies are a little more obliging:

She slept in a cot by our bed and whenever we had sex and I came – and I'm not noisy – she would wake up. There was such a strong tie between us. It would always make us laugh!

Sucked Dry by the Family

There are many complex emotional strands to parenthood, but one that women often find particularly hard to deal with is the sense of being sucked dry by everyone else's emotional needs, without having their own needs met. This can eliminate a woman's desire for sex:

I was used to having a healthy sexual appetite. But after my first baby was born I felt very exploited, by my husband and by the baby. I felt as if I had some other person on my body all the time. My breasts belonged to the baby; the other bits to my husband. I felt I had to carry out all my nurturing, maternal duties, yet I felt unable to say no to sex. In terms of needs and priorities I was at the bottom of the pile. I learned that resentment is the biggest passion killer.

We start having sex; he's saying 'I want you' – then you hear one of the children calling 'Mummy I want you!' And I have to say 'Hang on darling' (to them both), and then 'I'll bring dolly in a minute.' Sex and motherhood just doesn't mix.

I've done all the holding all day long. By the time we get to bed I just want to be held myself.

All day long I've been seeing to the needs of a baby and a toddler. I feed them, change them, play with them, comfort them, rock them to sleep. By the end of the day I need someone to be there for me, to look after me. But my husband comes home from work and either falls asleep in front of the telly, or wants me to turn him on. I prefer it when he falls asleep in front of the telly, because by the end of the day I just haven't got any more to give.

The months and years of new parenthood are a notorious roller coaster, sometimes heavenly, sometimes hellish. All of your emotional and physical resources are stretched to the limit. The baby absorbs endless amounts of love and attention. You sense that your partner also needs more from you. But meanwhile, who is giving *you* the support you need? This is a time when it can feel as if there simply isn't enough love to go around, and sex is often an early casualty.

What can you do? Enjoy the baby – and know that sex will start again in the long years you have ahead together. It feels like this is a time that lasts forever; it doesn't.

Now that my nights are longer – the children are sleeping through at last – my libido is gradually coming back. I feel now that I'm on a more equal footing with him. If he initiates sex, I'm quite happy.

He was pussyfooting around me for a long time, but we needed to really talk about it – in a way to ask each other's permission – before we could say yes. I'm grateful that he didn't pressurize me, and talking about it brought us a lot closer. Then, lo and behold, we had sex!

In the long term too, the whole experience of becoming parents can bring you closer in ways you could never predict. As Jane Hawksley puts it:

Sex always does get better later on when you've reached a level of ease with each other, that crucial risk-free area. That's what we come to really value; after your husband has seen you giving birth and he still loves you, the real you. That is a wonderful thing.

CHAPTER 4

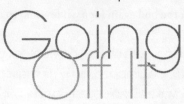

Going Off It

Whether it is the exhaustion of new parenthood or life's other myriad trials, there are plenty of reasons why sex sometimes sinks to the bottom of your agenda for a while. The first time this happens you may feel desperately worried:

When we were first married, if it got to the end of the week and we hadn't made love I would get really upset. When we were courting we sometimes used to do it two or three times in an afternoon – and then a couple of times after supper and again in the morning. So the first time we did nothing in an entire week, I was devastated!

But one of the great advantages of being in a long-term couple is that you've got *perspective*. You've probably been through a spell of celibacy before with your partner, so you know that your relationship isn't on the rocks just because you haven't done it for a few weeks – or even months.

For most long-term relationships are a matter of continuous ebb and flow. To begin with you can't wait to get into bed together; then you go 'off it' for a bit. All being well, desire returns, sex improves – and then goes off the boil again for a while – and so on:

I think the frequency with which you want sex varies throughout life. My own libido dropped away dramatically when I had the kids, and now it has increased again – but unfortunately, out of step with my husband's!

Some couples carry on having sex fairly regularly, but without the urgent, melting lust that once made it all so easy:

We have sex without kissing now, which never happens when you are in a new relationship.

Most of the time I don't initiate sex because it's not to the forefront of my mind. But once we get down to it, I do really enjoy it and I always end up thinking – we should do this more often!

- Reported frequency of heterosexual sex (vaginal, oral and anal) varies considerably with age, marital status and length of relationship.
- Women aged 20–29 and men aged 25–34, particularly if married or cohabiting, reported the highest average occurrence of five times per month.
- More than 50 per cent of women aged 55–59 reported no sex in the last month.

- Frequency of sex reduces as the length of a relationship increases. This occurs across all age groups, suggesting that declining sexual activity is not due entirely to age.

(From Factsheet No. 6, The Family Planning Association.)

Sometimes it seems as if you just can't have your cake and eat it; as if the price of a good relationship is not-so-good sex:

I used to think that as long as I had a good rogering every night, as long as we had great sex, everything in the relationship would be fine. I used to have great sex, but crap relationships. Now it's the other way around.

Sometimes there are deep and difficult reasons why desire dies in a relationship. Like buried anger. Like sadness. Like fear. These may stem from the murkier regions of a couple's relationship – such as their childhoods, their family backgrounds or their relationships with their own parents.

Some relationships reach such a peak of frustration and desperation that there is violence. Others sink into depression. Either way, the desire for sex is usually an early casualty.

After a series of major changes in their lives, Chris and her partner found themselves drifting apart:

We have been through a very difficult time recently and our sex life has just about ground to a halt. We recently tried to have sex again and it was great for him but not for me. That's because for me everything is coming from a place of fear;

how do I hang on to this relationship? It was desperation on my part. I feel tremendous love for him, but no desire.

As Anne explained in Chapter 1, she too went through a time of desperation and fear during which sex stopped all together:

At the time when we were having our difficulties Marcus was very angry and frustrated. The kids would be crying because of all the anger and verbal abuse and I felt I had to protect them. I felt very cold towards him in bed; I didn't even want him to touch me. We slept in separate rooms. It was an extremely hurtful time.

Yet, as we have seen, Anne and Marcus managed to resolve their difficulties and – it's no coincidence – rebuild their sex life.

Sometimes the loss of desire is a sign that there is no point in trying to stay in a relationship; it may be time to cut your losses and leave – or it may be time to get help. Relate counsellors and psychosexual therapists are trained to guide you through this particular minefield.

But the ordinary, day-to-day business of living with another person can be hell at times, and it's true that most couples do go through some seriously bad patches. Yet often – with love and a bit of open communication – things slowly improve, desire returns and sex becomes a vital expression of commitment once again:

I just didn't want to have sex when the children were very small. I felt – I've given all I'm prepared to give today. But it does come back. It does get better again. My kids are teenagers now and I have to shut myself up these days when I come, in case of what my neighbours might think.

In her personal account of her sexual relationship with her long-term partner, *Light My Fire*, author Arabella Melville charts their early passion – and its decline into boredom:

How it Began...

'Sex was simple and delightful...Our lust was intense. We would have sex anywhere, everywhere we could...(There were) two years when the nights we didn't make love were remarkable for their rarity. We didn't need elaborate fore-play; the very idea of sex was enough to turn us on. I was always available for him. Orgasm came quickly, easily, repeatedly.'

How it Became...

After 10 years of living together, it was a different story:

'In bed, as elsewhere, I was passive, often uninterested but unwilling to admit this even to myself. Colin (my part-ner), bewildered, attributed my lack of passion to my age... The pattern of my sex life was one of dominance and sub-mission. He decided how much foreplay there should be and when to penetrate me; if I wasn't ready, I didn't tell him. I was almost always underneath him, controlled by his weight. I wanted sex, because without it I felt rejected, neglected, undesirable, unloved; but I contributed little to

its success…We lived in a featureless landscape of boredom and unsatisfied needs.'

Why Oh Why Oh Why?

So why is it that – even when we feel our relationship is going well –
some of us simply seem to lose desire for sex? Loss of desire has
been called the 'disease of the 1990s', while surveys show that more
than a third of American women and one in six American men admit
to having lost their desire for sex.

- Shere Hite's *The Hite Report on Male Sexuality* reveals
  that men's greatest complaint about women is that they
  don't want as much sex as men do.
- Loss of libido is also the main reason why people con-
  sult a sex therapist, and it is known to be an important
  factor in heralding the breakdown of a relationship.
- The old, macho stereotype of the man who is 'always up
  for it' seems to be crumbling. The number of couples
  attending Relate clinics with difficulties attributed to
  lack of sexual desire in the man has almost doubled in
  the past few years. The most frequent complaint is now
  erection problems, very much linked to loss of desire.

Meanwhile, at the end of the 1990s, a series of newspaper and mag-
azine features seems to be suggesting that people – especially young
people – simply aren't particularly interested in sex these days.

'No Sex Please, We're Married', was the title of a story in *Vogue* (July 1996) about how many women are having to close their eyes and 'think of England'. Meanwhile the *Independent on Sunday* ran a feature headlined 'The Great Male Headache' which described how 'far from being sex-crazed beasts, more and more men are reporting sluggish libidos'.

Sex as the driving force for a relationship is out of fashion, as relationships psychologist and author Susan Quilliam told *The Independent on Sunday*:

There is a real feeling of choice among young people; a boy is not now desperate to prove he's a man by having sex. Young people are saying, 'We're not like our parents, who rushed into sex because they thought they couldn't have it; now we've got it we are going to put it in perspective.'

I think the push for men to want lots of sex was largely social, because it simply wasn't acceptable for women to make the first move. Now that has changed and sex drive is being more equally distributed. The onus is off men to make the first move, so they don't need to be as driven.

Bed and Bored?

So could it be that we are simply going off sex because we're sick of it? Has the so-called sexual revolution dished up so much of the stuff that we've simply lost our appetite? In his book *Rituals of Love* author Ted Polhemus argues that in making sex more open and possible (even mandatory), we have evaporated away its power:

In our contemporary frenzy of unlimited sex we have lost everything – eroticism, desire, even ironically, sex itself – because we have lost the frisson of the seductive. Like a supernova no longer able to sustain itself, our contemporary sexuality has imploded and emits no radiance because it possesses no magic, no poetry, no charm, no veiled illusion, no sorcery, no secrets and no playfulness.

Polhemus finds new 'magic' in the rituals of bondage, sado-masochism and the fetish scene – as do many couples in long-term relationships. But his view of lost lust is rather dramatic for all that: it's not as if we're a nation of celibates except for a sprinkling of rubber enthusiasts!

No, the vexed question of why desire fades is a complex one and many a theory has sprung up to explain it. There may well be truth in all of them.

MOVING ON

First of all, why *should* we expect to keep up the frantic level of sex which we once experienced in the 'courtship' phase of our relationships? Most of us don't expect to carry on doing the other things many of us did when we were in our teens or early 20s, like drinking and partying all night, like living as if we hadn't a care in the world – or, at least, not to the same extent.

'You can't sustain the exciting and spontaneous sex of the courtship phase,' argues sex therapist Jane Hawksley. 'You would be worn out.' The truth is simply that most of us move on and mature – mentally, emotionally and physically. Our lives become more complex and more committed. It's all very well being madly in lust and going at it all night long if you don't have to get up in the morning to go to work or to get children off to school, but generally speaking, adulthood brings responsibilities.

It may be essential in getting couples bonded, but urgent lust is hardly compatible with the long slow haul of bringing up children, earning a living and keeping a home together. There comes a time when it really is more important to get some sleep than to have sex.

Indeed, survey after survey has shown that in terms of marital happiness – for women – sexual satisfaction rates quite low. For men, it rates higher but it is still not their first priority. Far more important to most married couples is companionship.

So instead of harking back sentimentally to those days of automatic simultaneous ecstasy (was it always *really* that good?), let's face facts: we are grown-ups now, things have changed – and in many ways for the better. Sex may not be as frantic or as frequent, but for many long-term couples it gets more raunchy and more deeply satisfying with time (*see Chapter* 7).

As Jane Hawksley puts it:

There are compensations in a long-term relationship. You may lose out on spontaneity, but you have learned how to arouse each other. From a 'cold start' you know how to have very good sex.

Not Doing it Enough? Says Who?

Julia Cole of Relate has this to say:

'Couples often say to me – we only do it once a month, which is not enough. I say to them – but how do you feel about it?

'I try to give them the idea that if they feel okay about doing it once a month, then that's fine.

'They feel enormous relief at not having to fit in with what magazines and other media tell them is "normal".

'If you've got a young child, or you've just lost your job, or you are ill, or you have money worries, the last thing on your mind is sex. In situations like these you rightly need to put your emotional energies into the rest of your life.

If you have got a strong relationship, the sexual element will return. Most people say they go through periods when they make love a lot, and others when they don't bother – and still others when they show each other lots of affection.

'Although some people still think of sex as nothing but penetrative sex, I do remind people that the act of penetration is not "it"; a sexual relationship is a totality which has many other aspects.

'People are often scared of saying – "I do need you to hold me, but that may not lead to sex". But we can't do without affection in a relationship. It's very important to be able to laugh and put an arm around each other, to give each other a kiss on the cheek when we come home after work. As a therapist I am not so worried about how often people "do it"; it is more important to be able to do these other things.'

LIKE BROTHER AND SISTER

One intriguing theory about why desire fades is that we are biologically programmed *not* to be strongly sexually attracted to the people we live with. This has obvious benefits. It prevents all kinds of murder and mayhem within small communities – including that smallest of all communities, the family.

It is a fact that brothers and sisters who grow up together very rarely fall in love with each other. Instead they develop the kind of ultra-familiar, deeply loyal and comfortably bickering relationship which is remarkably like many marriages. Of course, most of us love our brothers and sisters very much – rather like our long-term partners – but the idea of going to bed with them doesn't enter our heads.

Women who have lived with the same male partner for many years can know just how that feels:

Once we'd moved in together all the charm and flowers gave way to this rather moody bloke who grunts at me from time to time and competes with me to get the comfiest chair or the biggest helping of food. There's only one other man in the world who is as close to me – and as grumpy with me – as my husband is, and that's my brother.

We still have our raunchy phases, but he's almost like my brother now. We've got such a close relationship that we've lost that sexual mystery of the stranger.

Yet studies of twins who have been separated at birth and brought up in different families indicate a remarkable phenomenon. In contrast to brothers and sisters who have grown up under the same roof, those who have grown up separately and who only meet each other for the first time as adults do quite often fall passionately in love.

Is this just a social taboo against incest, or is there some kind of subtle biochemical process going on here? Either way, couples who live together for many years find different ways – through fantasy, playing different roles, or just ringing the changes – to make things stimulatingly new again.

As Marcus put it in Chapter 1:

We are continually making adjustments in our lives – mostly to accommodate our children – so we have to be inventive. If our physical relationship didn't have to negotiate these changes it would probably come to an end through boredom. But because we are continually making these adjustments, it leads to variations in our lovemaking. Life imposes changes which keeps things alive between us.

TURNING INTO MUMMY?

Another major passion-killer – for many women at least – is the shift from being their man's lover to being his surrogate mum. We've seen how this can happen after the arrival of a baby, but it can also happen without them.

Chris, aged 32, has been going through a very difficult time with her husband of five years:

When his parents died he retreated into himself and slowed down. We had moved to be near his family home and I found that he continued to retreat. I feel that he is trying to re-create his childhood past with me in the role of 'mum'. I am expected to be in full caretaker mode; I am living a life that isn't mine.

My response has been to cut off from him sexually, partly as a way of putting up a barrier, partly as a way to challenge him to 'reclaim me'. I want to get out of this mother/child situation and return to being lovers and equals. I was trying to make a certain point by retreating, wanting him to claim me. But he has been quite happy not to take up the challenge. He just says politely, oh well, if that's the way you feel…He is disappointed and a bit frustrated – but he has made no effort to claim me.

But I only have one life. I am not going to give it up to be someone's caretaker. If 90 per cent of my energy goes into meeting his needs, how can I be fulfilled and creative and contribute something to the world?

I think there is a split for men between their 'wife' and their 'lover'. Before marriage it is easier for a man to see you as his 'lover', but once you've tied the knot you become a potential mother and so your desire is less acceptable. Especially after the death of his own mother I feel very 'maternalized'.

It is men's conditioning, but it makes me very angry. If I ever have a son I want to help him to have access to his emotions so that he can understand and express them. It is our job to bring up the next generation differently to avoid all this pain. I do still feel tremendous love for him, but no desire.

Sometimes it is the woman who takes on the role of mother in a relationship – to the puzzlement of her partner. But then we too are subject to conditioning, as Phillipa has discovered to her cost:

I was brought up to believe that food is very important and that women are there to provide it. And despite the fact that my career is important to me, from the time we started sharing a flat together I was rushing home at the end of the day to be 'mum'.

He is appalling in the kitchen and because I loved him I thought that if I didn't feed him he wouldn't eat healthy food. But by the time I'd finished the lasagne – or whatever – I'd be exhausted, and he'd eat and go down to the pub with his mates.

Then came a time when he was working and I went back to university. Because I wasn't paying as much towards our living expenses I felt that it was my place to keep the flat clean and get dinner on the table. I turned into a mother figure which did affect our relationship. A pattern of resentment built up. I hate confrontation so I would hold in my feelings, but inside I was thinking 'You can't even be bothered to cook some pasta: in that case I can't be bothered to go to bed with you!'

When we broke up we discussed what had happened and he told me that he had hated it. He wanted me to go to the pub with him to get slaughtered from time to time. I simply got mumsy too quickly; it was nice for a while but I turned into the Nurturing Person and he thought I was boring.

Fortunately there is a positive ending to Phillipa's story. After a year-long split with her man, they are back together again, and she says, 'very happy'. But they have learned from their mistakes: instead of living in stultifying domesticity with Phillipa playing mum, so far they are living apart but visiting each other on weekends with all the excitement of a new courtship.

'I like sex, but I don't need it any more...'

Many women do become mothers (*see Chapter 4*), which affects us at the deepest emotional level, with huge implications for our sexuality. Sarah has been married for over 10 years, and in that time the deep needs which once drove her sexual desire have changed:

'My partner keeps harking back to the time when we first got together; when I was passionately in love with him and sex was always spontaneously, orgasmically wonderful.

'Things have changed; of course they have. We met at a time in my life when I had no-one – except for friends and boyfriends. I had left my family – I no longer had a home – and no regular source of love and affection. Naturally, I craved love. I was absolutely driven to find a mate to establish a new home, a new identity. Looking for that mate was a wonderful, desperate, terrifying, exciting roller-coaster ride.

'And then I found him. It was bliss! For a few years. Then came the first baby. Then the second, and the third. I had little bodies clinging to me, climbing onto my lap for years on end: no shortage of love and affection. They wrap their arms around your neck, tell you they love you.

'Before going to bed at night I always check they are alright. There they are, sleeping peacefully, looking so beautiful. I put my cheek on theirs; I kiss them goodnight. My heart is full of love for them; I feel so lucky.

'Next stop: our bedroom. Poor man, what can he offer me which compares with that? How can he ever be as gorgeous? How can he compete?

'Sex has now become an optional extra in my life. It's a pleasure I can take or leave. I don't need it any more.'

CALLING TIME ON LOVE AND LUST

Another interesting theory is that Nature never intended us to live so long with one other partner. In fact, Nature may not have intended us to live so long at all. It's a remarkable fact that we in the West now live nearly twice as long as people did during the many thousands of years which precede us. It follows that our relationships may go on for decades, a situation unprecedented in human history.

'Most divorces take place five to nine years after the wedding,' says Julia Cole of Relate, a time span long enough to start a new family. 'The first baby is the biggest hurdle in most relationships. We have to cope with enormous change, reinventing ourselves, moving from being partners to being parents as well. If our relationship survives, it may be stronger in the long term, but it may not feel like that at the time.'

According to the Office of National Statistics, the average length of a settled relationship these days is nine years. Historically, the average length of a marriage was about the same. In the past, there were so many plagues, wars and deaths in childbirth that most husbands and wives simply died before they had time to start worrying about their loss of lust.

It's surely no coincidence that we talk about the 'seven-year itch' as a time of restless dissatisfaction which can set in seven years after a marriage. Add that to – perhaps – a two-year courtship, and we're back to that figure of nine years.

Contrast the situation of many couples today who are together for four or five times that long, long enough for four or five different 'nine-year' relationships. Look at long-term relationships in this light and is it any wonder that desire sometimes flags?

Instead of beating ourselves up with worry that we aren't in a state of permanent lust for each other, perhaps we should be congratulating ourselves on surviving a long voyage into territory hitherto unexplored by the human race!

LIBERATED WOMEN, INSECURE MEN?

One of the implications of living with someone for a long period of time is that both of you are going to develop and change. In many ways we are not the same people at 30 or 40 as we were at 20. Time rubs off our rough edges, sharpens our priorities and can boost – or damage – our self-esteem.

For women especially, life falls into distinct time zones – because we are still the ones who take on most of the burden of care for children, and later in life for elderly relatives. Some women hate it when the time comes for children to leave home, suffering from the 'empty nest syndrome' with all its accompanying depression and low libido (*see Further Reading in Resources*).

But many women find that, on the contrary, their 40s and 50s are a time of great rejuvenation. At last they are free of the constraints of young children; at last they can get back to the mainstream, get a job, get on with all they have put on the back burner for so long.

The Shifting Balance of Power

- 75 per cent of young women feel able to rear their children without the necessity of a male breadwinner.
- One in five women now earns more than her male partner (compared with one in 15 a decade ago).

(Source: 'Freedom's Children', Demos survey into attitudes of 18–34 year olds.)

For men, however, this great resurgence of energy can feel more as if 'her indoors' is suddenly straining at the leash. 'Women have been through feminism with all the changes that implies,' says Julia Cole of Relate, 'whereas men can still be quite fearful of those changes. They are told they can't be macho any more – yet women also want them to be more decisive. Sometimes they just don't know what they are supposed to be.'

Inevitably, this has its repercussions in the bedroom. In his play about a relationship in crisis, *LOVEBITES*, Tom Clark, founder of the Gog Theatre Company, writes about the tensions which can develop between men and women in the wake of feminism:

MAN: Are you having an affair? Look at me!

WOMAN: If that's what you want to make sense of things. Affair or no affair, it makes no difference. The hour has come. One of us is going to walk.

MAN: What really hurts is your dishonesty. Your closed legs for the feminist cause. Why couldn't you just say: 'Honey, I've fallen out of love, sorry'. Sex; you fear its domination. Me on top, you become a traitor to your beliefs. Is that it? You women are in danger of turning your juices into ink for your printing presses and soon you'll be all dry inside, as dry as the pages of your fragmented, confused manifestos.

I don't know where I stand any more. Men don't know where they lie even in their own beds.

And in another scene:

WOMAN: I'm your woman. W.O.M.A.N. To have and to hold. To have me, to hold me, to stick it in.

Stuck with you...and endless love? A fairytale where you could see yourself in me and me in you. It's not endless for anyone.

I've done enough. Now it's my turn. I want a life.

I'm not your emotional insurance scheme. Never satisfied with yourself – expect me to provide you with the missing pieces.

Cutting Loose: a Man's Point of View

James went through a crisis in his marriage which he believes was linked to his wife's growing need for freedom as their children became less dependent upon her:

'When the kids don't really need a woman any more, she's off. A huge shift takes place. Suddenly, there's no need for her to organize what we would all do every weekend. It was – What do I do? What's my function now? It accelerated really fast and you could see the glue of our relationship just melting.

'I found her diary where she had written that our sex life was of no interest to her. She accused me of invading her privacy, but she said it was the truth.

'It's this "call" that comes to a woman as soon as she feels free of her infants. You hear odd stories about other couples, but you don't know anything until it happens. This is the primordial drive of the 40-plus woman. She was nourished and fed socially and politically by the women's movement which was calling and calling her to cut loose.

'I missed her terribly. I'd ring and say – Don't you miss me? And she'd say – No, not at all. All this stuff about dependency: the man becomes like a child.'

LIFE AND DEATH ISSUES

Even when you seem to be getting on very well, life has a habit of butting in and spoiling everything – including your sex life. You or your partner might suddenly lose your job. Money worries can escalate into daily and nightly mental torture. Health problems can strike, making you doubt your future and even your attractiveness. Anxiety and depression are big-league passion-killers.

The death of someone close to you can also play havoc with a happy, healthy sex life:

The death of my mother drove us apart because my husband was afraid that I would go off the rails. It made him withdraw from me at a time when I needed him most.

After my mother died we went through a period of abstinence from August to the February of the next year. That was
how the grieving process worked in me. My brother told me,
however, that it got to him in quite the opposite way, and that
he was like a rabbit for months.

Grief and bereavements from the past can also cast a long shad-
ow over current sexual relationships:

I still can't stand my husband going away from me. I think that's
because of the death of my father. I went to work on a normal
day, and by that night he was dead. It was the saddest thing
and it screwed me up for quite a long time. My response for a
while was to chuck all my boyfriends before they could chuck
me. I never really said goodbye to my father. It's taken me 25
years to see what an effect that had on my sexual relationships.

My father died when I was a child. It's like unfinished business:
a man has left you. After that I wanted to be the one in control
of any relationship and I pushed a lot of people away.

My husband says I am still like an angry child a lot of the time.
When we went to Relate for marriage guidance counselling I
ended up talking about my Dad.

On the other hand, a sudden bereavement can sometimes stop
you in your tracks, making you reassess the value of your relationship – with very positive results:

After the death of a friend recently, we made love twice in a week, which is unusual for us these days. It was very necessary somehow. We needed to bond closer, to show each other that we love each other.

After my father died, I needed to have sex with my partner with a need I hadn't experienced for years. I was very close to my father and I felt a tremendous emotional gap when he had gone. I drew closer to my partner, partly for comfort, partly to fill that gap.

Death throws everything into a different perspective. It can be so sudden and senseless that you want to draw everyone around you. There is an urgency to unite under the threat of death.

BUT IS SEX REALLY NECESSARY?

There is another – and totally heretical – way of looking at the loss of desire, and that is to shrug your shoulders and say 'No more sex? So what's the problem?' Rare though it is to suggest this in our sex-obsessed culture, not everybody actually *minds* not having sex. Lots of people don't have sex and yet live satisfying, interesting lives.

Sometimes, it's a relatively short period of celibacy:

A lot depends on how long you've been together. We've been together for 10 years and there were stretches of weeks, even months, when we went without sex. Yet it didn't seem to be a problem.

When we first met we were at it all the time, like a pair of rabbits. But after a few years we just seemed to lose our drive for it, and we went for weeks on end without even touching each other.

Celibacy, even for a short time, can be a positive choice. As Laura, aged 30, puts it:

When I was celibate I felt powerful. I took a step back and looked at this thing 'sex' that drives everybody. As a celibate person I was completely in control of my own life.

Sometimes, for complex reasons, celibacy is a permanent but not unhappy state. Sarah has been married for nearly 30 years to a man she loves very much. They have three children and a happy family life. Their relationship, however, has been a sex-free zone for the past decade:

I was 20 when I first met David. I thought he was lovely; very gentle. Was it 'love at first sight'? There was certainly something between us at first sight, and it was love – but not passion. We started going out together.

Soon after that I started living with him and we started having sex, but we treated it as something to laugh about. I was more marauding, more highly sexed than him. After a while our level of desire became equal and we didn't do it very often.

I was desperate to marry him. I loved him and I felt very right with him; safe and comfortable. We got married when I was 21 and we just adored each other.

The early years of our marriage were beset by extreme anxieties about my family who were going through a very bad patch, and during that time we experienced a lot of sexual problems. David had great difficulties with impotence. It had been a problem from the beginning and we both worried about it. We thought we should be doing it about four times a week, otherwise there was something 'abnormal' about us. We went to our GP who sent us to a specialist. It was so humiliating for David that we decided we'd just work it out in our own way.

As well as impotence, he also had a problem with premature ejaculation. But as he wasn't torturing himself about it, it seemed okay. We were best friends; a bit like brother and sister but without the incest taboo.

Looking back, I think we were attracted to each other because, sexually, we were a good fit. Neither of us was going to make demands that the other couldn't fulfil. I'd lost interest in sex after my initial randiness. These days we don't have sex with each other and we don't want to. In my 30s I faced the fact that I am sexually attracted to women and have had several love affairs with David's knowledge and consent.

We are such a close couple that if it is alright with us, the rest of the world can just go away. We have a lot of physical closeness and I feel that we always will have. Ours is a verbally and physically affectionate relationship and we tell each other that we love each other, so perhaps there is nothing more to be communicated through sex.

He says he likes everything about his life and that he is very happy as he is. I don't think we need sex with each other, and we have successfully resisted the outside pressures which decreed we should all be having lots of it.

For Better or for Worse...

For better or for worse, however, most of us *do* want to have a lively and continuing sex life with our partners over as many years as we've got. For sex is not just very good fun. At the very least, the tension that flows from sexual frustration can sabotage our domestic life, making us snappy and irritable with each other.

Sex can also be a kind of truce which descends on the age-old war between men and women, a time when the battleground of our often competing needs and power imbalances can become a place of mutuality and reconciliation.

And at best, sex can be a kind of transcendence which lifts us out of ourselves, unites us with our beloved and reaffirms all the reasons why we have chosen to commit ourselves to each other.

Sex matters to our sense of self too: many couples feel valued by each other when they are having an active sex life, because it means a lot to feel that you are still attractive to your partner. In many ways, sex is the glue that holds us together in spite of all that life may throw at us along the way.

CHAPTER 5

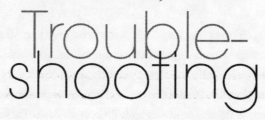

Trouble-shooting

However strong and satisfying our relationships can be, most of us find that sex in the long haul is not always plain sailing.

This chapter looks at five classic difficulties which can crop up simply because we don't all have the same needs and preferences, and because we change, slowly but surely, over time.

It also gives some suggestions and advice on how to handle these situations, which are:

1) You want sex when your partner doesn't – or vice versa.
2) You want your partner to be loving before you make love. Your partner just wants to 'do it'.
3) You are often too tired even to think about it…
4) You are bored in bed (much as you hate to admit it).
5) You simply don't have time. Work and/or family life seem to have taken over.

1. Only One of You is Keen

You love each other and know you want to be together. All that you care about most in life, you share: your home, your values, your hopes and – for many couples – your children. You have your ups and downs, but fundamentally you feel you are right for each other except for one thing: one of you feels little or no desire for sex.

The stereotype of the woman with a headache suggests that women are usually the ones who 'go off it', but the reality is that either partner can experience loss of libido.

Michael is 36:

We have virtually everything anyone could want, from an affectionate relationship and two beautiful daughters, to good jobs and a lovely home. Everything is just as we would wish – apart from sex. Every now and then it rears its ugly head like a kind of monster which lives under our bed. It has the power to savage our relationship and leave us in tatters. The problem is that she wants it and I simply don't.

Louise is 30:

At university I had masses of casual sex, although I didn't enjoy it much. I never had an orgasm. I used to have sex out of desperation, to 'keep my man'. I was always wondering if this person would be THE ONE?

But now at last I am very happy; I am with someone who actually *likes* me.

There's just one problem: no sexual fireworks. We don't do it more than once a month and I still haven't had an orgasm. Whenever we do have sex it's because I want to have a baby. Am I normal? Is it right? Everything else in our relationship is fantastic. But I wonder – should I be with someone else?

Richard is 28:

My girlfriend would be up for it almost every night, but it's me who's usually tired and not feeling like it. Sex is good fun so it's a shame not to have more of it, but sometimes I just feel totally knackered. It's partly my job; partly the result of having a few pints and staying up too late.

Paula is 35:

Much as I hate to admit it, my libido seems to have been in retreat for some time now. We've been together for 10 years, and in the early days we were both at it hammer and tongs. I was as keen as he was, and if he didn't make love to me night and morning I would feel terribly rejected and upset, not to mention frustrated. But these days it always seems to be him that takes the initiative, and it takes him a lot longer to get me in the mood. It worries me that I'm not the woman I used to be, and it frustrates him that it all seems to be such hard work.

Sometimes, as with Richard, this imbalance of desire is not a very serious problem. In his case, humour and understanding are enough to get him through – and besides, on occasions it's his girlfriend who's too tired.

But a major difference in levels of desire can cause havoc in a relationship – because the reasons for it often go deep.

'My experience is that an imbalance in desire suggests a problem in the relationship,' says Julia Cole of Relate, 'and it usually points to feelings of anger or disappointment, or the issue of control. It could be about feeling overwhelmed by a needy partner; it could be anger over a past event such as an affair; it could be a matter of one person feeling controlled, or needing to be in control.'

In other words, a loss of interest in sex can be a physical response to emotional pain. (It can also be a simply biological problem: *see Helpful Organizations in Resources*). Sometimes, of course, there are no deep or buried emotional traumas: just the simple fact that one partner is more interested in sex than the other.

Reluctant Women?

'It is a myth that men are keener than women to have sex,' believes Jane Hawksley, who has been a psychosexual therapist for 25 years. 'Men get erections all the time; it's nothing to them, whereas women feel that they have to take care of that erection. But male arousal is so quick; the penis can go up and down like a yo-yo. Women's arousal, on the other hand, is much slower, and its effects last for a much longer time.'

So how should we respond to these differences? Many couples want to 'balance up' their libidos, says Julia Cole:

But why should our sexual needs be the same? And why are couples keen for them to be the same? Does she want to shut him up – or does he want to control her? When she gives in, will he feel 'I've got what I wanted'? Or when she doesn't, will she feel 'I'm keeping a bit of myself back'?

If the answer to these questions is 'yes', it's worth looking closely at the relationship to see what makes it tick, believes Julia Cole.

Hot Tip: Make a Deal

It may sound a bit cold-hearted – because we prefer to think of sex and love as magically spontaneous – yet in reality most relationships are a kind of 'deal'. Unless we get what we want, and give what our partner needs, we are going to have problems – and the sexual arena is no exception.

So if you feel that your partner's 'demands' are putting you under pressure, why not negotiate? That way you can get what you both want without just waiting for it to happen – and if it makes you both happy, what's wrong with that?

You will have to think about what you want (not easy, especially for women) and what you can give. You'll also have to put it into words!

Make sure you both feel you are getting a fair deal. It will be more fun than you might think!

The Currency of Sex: Five 'Deals'

Trade   dressing up in that kinky outfit
For   giving or receiving oral sex.

Trade   saying out loud what you want during sex
For   an afternoon quickie.

Trade   doing it once or twice during the week as well
         as on weekends
For   doing it more slowly.

Trade   massage with scented oils
For   a candlelit dinner.

Trade   telling him/her your fantasies
For   starting earlier, taking longer.

'ASK WHY? AND NEGOTIATE...'

Psychosexual therapist Jane Hawksley takes a very practical and positive approach to the problem of loss of desire in one partner. In her view, honest communication is the key, and she makes these recommendations:

- Ask yourselves – why are we not making love, and what are we going to do about it? Why are we putting sex on the back burner? It's about getting to the truth.
- Say how you really feel; no excuses.
- If you don't want sex, *negotiate*. Say 'I'll have a cuddle with you, but not this or that'. Say 'I do love you and this is what I can give you'.

- Discuss what it is that turns you off. Does he or she come in after work and grope you without preamble? Does he or she sit watching telly with growing resentment, waiting for you to make the first move? Are you angry about the socks he leaves on the bedroom floor? Or about money? Or about who takes care of the kids? These are changeable things which you can work on.
- Always start with 'I', not 'you'. Say calmly how you feel and your partner can respond without going off the deep end. Don't make accusations, or he or she will respond in kind.

Says Jane Hawksley:

If you can't give him sex, then do the mothering bit for a while – but not ad infinitum – to tide you over. Cook him his favourite meal. After all, men are very simple creatures, easily pleased. They don't expect much. Why should we balk at these simple strategies? All this may sound rather brutal, but there are a lot of exasperated men around (and it is usually men) who are saying women want them to do everything when it comes to sex. They say they've got a headache or they've got a period, when what they are really saying is 'I don't feel like it'.

Training Your Man

'Men are very good at courtship,' believes Jane Hawksley, 'because they have got a goal to work towards. But once a relationship is up and running it is usually women who are good at maintaining it. If a man is getting regular sex and food on the table – and if there is a certain amount of domestic harmony – he is unlikely to rock the boat. It tends to be women who want to improve things.

'But it's important to be subtle and not go at things hammer and tongs. And it's no good saying "I wish you'd be nice to me" – but without reciprocating in any way. Women sometimes want all the courtship without any of the sexy bits.

'People only do things if they are going to gain by it. Men could get a livelier sex life if they did the things that needed doing! You can train men, but you have to do it in subtle ways; we can change men, but on their own terms. Men will go along with things if there is a reward for them.'

TAKING UP POSITIONS

Another issue for long-term couples is how we take on opposite roles in our relationships. As Marcus explained in Chapter 1, it happens in the rest of our lives – she cooks, I wash up; she vacuums, I cut the grass – and it happens in sex too.

No matter how close we are at the start, it doesn't take long for one of us to become the one who starts things off in bed, while the other waits for the advances.

If this becomes a habit, sex can become a problem. For sex is not just a love game; it can be a power game too.

Some men complain they always have to make the first move – but when *she* makes the first move, they can't handle it. American sex therapist Dagmar O'Connor, author of *How to make love to the same person for the rest of your life* (*see Further Reading in Resources*), describes a couple, Louis and Brenda, who came to see her after a year-long stretch of celibacy.

For 14 years, Louis had been making the first move while Brenda – usually – acceded. But one night, after Brenda had had a few drinks at a party, she reached under the bedclothes and began to caress Louis.

Far from being delighted, Louis pushed her hand away and accused her of being drunk. He said he didn't want to make love to her – because she didn't seem like herself. Brenda was angry; Louis was baffled.

Dagmar O'Connor points to a classic male attitude: that women are either Madonnas (good and pure, wife material) or 'whores' (sexy but sluttish, lover material). Louis, she suggested, couldn't handle the idea of his wife being 'sluttish' in the marriage bed.

Furthermore, it was not just Brenda's inhibitions which had kept her sexual urges locked in; her husband *wanted* them kept locked in! 'Initiation Rights' were his and his alone. Brenda paid him back by refusing sex herself the next time he made advances. Their sex life ground to a halt.

POWER GAMES

But Dagmar O'Connor doesn't leave it there. Why did Brenda put up with the imbalance in their situation for so long? What was in it for her? she asks. The answer she comes up with is another 'right', the 'Right of Refusal'. Brenda herself had exercised an ancient form of power, used by women the world over. The power to say 'no':

Traditionally, this 'Right of First Refusal' has been a woman's source of sexual power going back to her earliest sexual experiences. In almost all cases, she was the one who unilaterally decided with whom and when she lost her virginity. And in most marriages, she has retained this control ever since. She rations sex. It is her prime unit of exchange. When she 'gives in' she is entitled to her husband's gratitude, and perhaps even some favour. And when she refuses his sexual advances she is 'keeping him in line', letting him know who is the ultimate sexual boss.

A starkly primitive view of sex? Well, sex can be a pretty primitive business. In most marriages, writes O'Connor:

It is still the man who actively initiates sex the majority of the time. And it is still the woman who maintains the right of refusal. Time and again women come to my office complaining that they do not enjoy sex only to discover that they are unwilling to enjoy sex because if they did they would relinquish their sexual control over their mates. A woman who actively enjoys sex can no longer claim to be giving in.

There is a happy ending to the Brenda and Louis story. Dagmar O'Connor got them to pelt each other with ping pong balls in the nude to vent their anger, and then, after a range of touching exercises, to take turns at initiating sex. Their sex life was soon back on track with Louis joking that Brenda still had to pay him back – for 14 years of making the first move!

Which begs the question – can there be equality in sex? Perhaps there can, when there is also equality in power between the sexes. Roll on, oh happy day!

2. Be Loving Before Making Love

It's a chicken-and-egg situation of love and lust: which comes first? Women, on the whole, tend to want emotional intimacy and tenderness before they feel like sex. Men, on the whole, like it the other way around.

After a row, too, women tend to want to make up before they make love again, whereas men often want to make love to make up…

Carol, 37, finds herself in this situation time and time again:

It usually follows a few days, sometimes as long as a week, in which we haven't had sex. Mind you, we have plenty of good reasons for not having sex – like being too preoccupied with work, or falling out over something.

But the tension seems to build from there. We become increasingly ratty and exasperated with each other. The atmosphere in the house is heavy with little jibes and short remarks.

The sad thing is that he just wants me to spontaneously want him; but how can I when he is angry and sulking because – evidently – I don't. It's catch-22.

Eventually we get around to talking. What is going on, we ask each other? He then obliquely refers to the fact that life isn't much fun these days. I know he is saying that he is unhappy that our sex life seems to be on hold, and I know he is saying he would like me to do something to turn him on. 'See you later,' he'll say hopefully, on his way out of the door to work. 'Perhaps you could surprise me tonight!'

But that leaves me feeling totally exasperated because what he is saying is that he needs me to be someone other than me – in order to fancy me. He doesn't want to be with the needy, stressed-out me who wants him to put an arm around me, just to show he cares. Instead he wants me reinvented as some rampaging sex pot. Then he will be very attentive to me indeed.

I want him to sit down with me as I really am, show me some affection and support, be nice to me for a while. But I know that in order to 'make things better' – as he sees it – I'm going to end up attending to his needs first. Sometimes it feels as if we are like two children in need of love and affection, but there just isn't enough of it to go around. I need it from him – but he needs it from me.

Usually, with a bit of prompting from him, I do make the effort; we do have sex – and the tension lifts. If it was good, he wants to do it again the next night and the next night, until something happens – we have an argument, or I get my period – sex goes on hold again, and we're back to being irritable with each other.

It is a truth universally acknowledged that sex can mean different things to men and women. As Denise Knowles of Relate puts it:

To a man it often means 'I'll show you how much I love you by making love to you'. But to women it has other implications. Women tend to say 'I need to feel love before I make love'. Women have more of a hidden agenda.

The roots of all this lie very deep. Things have started to shift in recent decades, but historically, across the globe, women have been obliged to take second place to men. These fundamental issues of power and status reverberate in the bedroom. 'Time and again in counselling we hear that women are not feeling valued enough outside of the bedroom,' says Denise Knowles. 'They feel as if men consider them to be sex objects.'

The issue is further complicated by the fact that men and women do have different ways of communicating. 'Men often don't feel comfortable about showing their emotions,' according to Denise Knowles. 'For them, sex is an acceptable way to express their feelings.'

A MAN AND HIS PENIS

'For a lot of men the way to make up an argument is to make love,' says psychosexual therapist Jane Hawksley. 'On the other hand, women want to talk first, settle their disagreements – before they can make love. But women tend not to understand the relationship between a man and his penis. From boyhood onwards his penis is his friend and his comfort. When he wants to make love to settle a row, he is putting out his hand of friendship to you in perhaps the only way he can. So don't overreact and say "there you go again!" because he won't understand it.'

MIND YOUR LANGUAGE!

Understanding. Communication. Language. Are men really from Mars and women from Venus, both missing the point of what the other has to say? If so, we need to peel away many layers of 'meaning' from sex and get back to basics.

How many words or expressions do we have in our language for this incredibly complex act? As Rachel put it in Chapter 1:

Sex. Making Love. Fucking. We have only a handful of words to express these things, and that is not enough.

How do you put in words the kind of connection you have with someone else when sexual intercourse isn't about love at all – even when you are doing it with someone you have loved for many years?

Mary, aged 43, had a try:

We row a lot in our relationship, and from quite early on I noticed something quite disturbing. For me, anger is a turn-on. After a good shout and a lot of indignation, I feel very hot – in more ways than one. If we go to bed after – or during – a row we have great sex. It's as if I am a pressure cooker and orgasm lets out some of my steam! So we don't call this making love; that's far too soppy for what we do when we're angry! It's more a matter of 'fuck you mate!'

Dagmar O'Connor, sex therapist and author, calls it 'making anger'. She describes how she counselled a woman client to get on top of her man and do her worst, as it were, every time he suggested they 'hit the sack' after a row. O'Connor reckons that our romantic, idealized notions of love and marriage are the enemies of good sex. Sex can't always be 'meaningful' she argues; it's far more complicated and varied than that.

Take the case of Cherrill, aged 37. She describes herself as happily married to a solicitor, Mark. They have two children:

I get terribly worried if Mark is late getting home from work. Rationally I know that he is probably stuck in a meeting and can't get away to phone me. But the feeling of fear mounts and mounts, and before long it turns into anger. How can he do this to me, I rage. How dare he leave me without the courtesy of a phone call or message?

The anger builds up in me and I feel it as sexual tension. One evening while I was waiting for him – late again – I sat straddling the arm of the sofa, and as I rocked myself backwards and forwards feeling very agitated, I had an orgasm. Then another and another. In the half hour before he finally opened the front door I must have come about 20 or 30 times.

Of course, hidden anger and resentment can also be a major turn-off, and the best way to tackle these feelings is usually to discuss and express them openly. Having sex as a way of placating someone, papering over the cracks in a relationship, rarely works – at least not for long.

But all relationships – especially long-term ones – are very complex, encompassing a whole range of emotions. Romantic love is only one of those; 'making love' is only one kind of sex. There are plenty of others you could try, for instance:

- Silly sex – the kind where you tickle each other, wrestle naked, hit each other with pillows and collapse into helpless laughter.

- Falling asleep sex – when it's too late to finish what you've started.
- Revive 45 sex – the kind you have for old time's sake.
- Zipless sex – the Erica Jong variety, pure lust with no strings.
- 'Dry' sex – frenzied and (almost) fully clothed, so that technically you haven't done it at all.
- VSI – Vigorous Sexual Intercourse, very good for hangovers.
- Kinky sex – whatever turns you on…
- 'Fuck you mate' sex – rampant with rage.
- French film sex – when you've been to an erotic movie.
- The Big Tease – start what you don't intend to finish – until later.
- Command performance – when domination is your thing.
- Al fresco sex – an open-air sex picnic.

WHY MEN WANT SEX AND WOMEN DON'T:
WHAT THE SHRINKS SAY

Many women in long relationships go through times when sex is the last thing on their minds – often to the great frustration of their male partners. There are plenty of obvious reasons for this – like tiredness – but could there also be deeper reasons hidden in the mysteries of the female psyche?

If you want to know more about what the professionals have to say about this, a good place to start is Lillian B. Rubin's book *Intimate Strangers (see Further Reading in Resources)*. She puts forward a psychoanalytical explanation for why many women in long-term relationships avoid sex. This is based on the theory that our earliest childhood experiences of mothering shape our sense of self very profoundly so that girls grow up with a very different sense of their 'boundaries' than boys.

Unlike boys, Rubin argues, girls never have to define themselves as fundamentally different from their mothers because they are the same gender. As a result, women grow up with less clear 'ego boundaries' than men who, in contrast, have to cut themselves off emotionally from their first love ('mother') to identify themselves as male.

In this book many women have talked about feeling that – after a day spent at the beck and call of other people, often children – they have to protect their fragile sense of self from yet another invasion. Sex can seem like another 'demand' in their already overloaded lives.

According to Rubin this is because:

With entry (penetration), her boundaries have been violated, her body invaded. It's just this that may explain why a woman so often avoids the sexual encounter – a common complaint in marriages – even when she will also admit to finding it pleasurable and gratifying once she gets involved. For there is both pleasure and pain – the pleasure of experiencing the union, the pain of the intrusion that violates her sometimes precarious sense of her own separateness. Together, these conflicting feelings often create an inertia about sex – not about an emotional connection but about a sexual one – especially when she doesn't feel as if there's enough emotional pay-off in it to make it worth the effort to overcome her resistance to stirring up the conflict again.

Rubin's theory also offers an explanation for why some men seem to be so much more driven to have sex than women. Boys' upbringing (and she makes the assumption that women generally care for small children) leaves them with a 'split' between their emotions and their sexual desires. The emotional side of men's attachment to their mothers comes under attack at an early age, she believes, as boys have to 'repress' their identification with their mothers. But the erotic side of their natures – the sexual aspect of their love for their mothers – remains unaffected (in heterosexual men).

Writes Rubin:

This split between the emotional and the erotic components of attachment in childhood has deep and lasting significance for the ways in which we respond to relationships – sexual and otherwise – in adulthood. It means that, for men, the erotic aspect of any relationship remains forever the most compelling, while, for women, the emotional component will always be the more salient.

This also explains why women's (non-sexual) friendships are so important to them, whereas men tend to have far less emotional connection with people – unless there is a sexual connection too. For men, sex is the one area where our culture says it is okay for them to be in touch with their emotions. Perhaps this explains why men get so grumpy (according to their womenfolk) when sex is on the back burner. It's not so much a physical urge as a deep emotional urge that can only be expressed physically.

Hot Tips: When Things are Getting Tense

- Don't let the problem build. Nip it in the bud with physical affection, hugs and kisses. It is very difficult to stay angry with someone who is making you feel good.
- Break the vicious circle by going out with friends. We all tend to behave better in the company of other people – which gives you a chance to see afresh each other's charm, intelligence and wit!
- Talk and listen, listen and talk. If you can do it, it's the best way to get close again. After all, you both really want the same thing – you're just having trouble getting there.
- Have a drink, have a laugh, have a row – but whatever you do, have it out with each other.

3. Too Tired to Tango?

Another issue which can cause a great deal of tension in long-term relationships is the vexed question of sleep. Our needs for sleep can vary tremendously; some people do quite well on four or five hours, while others need a full eight or nine hours just in order to function.

Match a heavy sleeper with an insomniac, and no matter how much they love each other, there's going to be trouble. Throw a wakeful baby into the equation and it's likely to be hell on wheels for some time to come.

Tracy and Howard are in their mid-30s. They have a toddler and a baby. They both work. Tracy hasn't had an unbroken night's sleep for over a year:

Tracy:

There's never enough time in the day to do everything, what with work and children and keeping the house in order. So by the end of the day I'm pretty tired and yet by the time we can settle down and relax it's always after 10. We watch telly or read the paper for a while, and before we know it it's about half past 11 at night. It's usually me who gets up from the sofa and says – time for bed, are you coming up?

He looks a bit keen, so I say 'hurry up then' and head off up the stairs.

I get into bed and wait for him. And wait for him. But soon my eyelids are drooping, and if I don't hear him on the stairs, I can't help it, I drop off to sleep.

Next thing I know he's crept into bed beside me and his hands are all over me. But I don't feel very good tempered when I've just been woken up, and all I want to do is push him away. So he turns over in a sulk and I turn over feeling really cross – sometimes too cross to get back to sleep again.

Howard:

Why is she so tired all the time? She usually goes to bed a bit before me, but I'm only 10 or 15 minutes behind her and when I get into the bedroom, there she is, all bundled up like a dormouse snoring away. It's not exactly sexy is it?

It happens even when we go away on holiday. I go upstairs after a really enjoyable day and there she is, out for the count. It's not as if I'm a top priority. Sometimes it feels as if sex with me hasn't even made it onto her agenda!

COUPLE'S COUNSEL

There's not a lot you can do to change the amount of sleep you need, or the fact that you have a demanding job and/or family. But there are ways to handle things better, like saying 'no' politely (*see page 109*); like making a determined effort to go to bed earlier – even if one of you gets up again after you've had sex, leaving the other to sleep.

There would be no problem, of course, if we didn't think of bed-time and bed as the time and the place for sex. So why not try:

- ANOTHER TIME: making love at lunchtime – or any other time when you are at home together apart from at night.
- ANOTHER PLACE: making love somewhere other than the place where you sleep. In summer, take a rug into the great out-doors (don't get caught). Or make the most of other rooms where you live; bathrooms are a popular option. Sofas and arm-chairs are relatively comfortable. And then afterwards, go upstairs to bed and zzzzzzzzzz…
- ANOTHER SLEEP: if you are tired because of young children who wake you up in the night, try to get an afternoon nap (sleep when the baby sleeps), or a break from the children (could your own parents step in for a day or two?). You could also suggest to your partner that if you could have a few early nights to catch up – or lie-ins in the morning – it might eventually be worth his while!

There are practical changes you can make too, so that one of you doesn't get far more tired than the other:

1) SHARE THE BURDEN: it remains a sad fact that housework is shared equally in only one per cent of homes in the UK, and women are still the chief childcarers, especially for small children. It doesn't take a genius to work out why many women complain of tiredness. A little more equality on the home front can mean a lot more equality in bed.

2) LOOK AFTER YOUR HEALTH: many recent mothers suffer from a low level of anaemia, making them all the more weary. It may be worth asking your doctor to give you a blood test and, if necessary, taking a course of iron.

3) SOUND MIND, SOUND BODY: a healthy and nutritious, balanced diet goes a long way towards combating fatigue. Steer clear of too much alcohol (more than a couple of glasses of wine will send most tired people straight to sleep). Nicotine also keeps you awake, so if you must smoke, have your last fag at least half an hour before you want to be asleep. Caffeine is the enemy of refreshing rest; avoid tea and coffee late in the day and try camomile instead.

4) FIT FOR ANYTHING: regular exercise will not only make you feel more relaxed and energetic but it will also keep you in better shape for taking your clothes off. If aerobic exercise is not for you, yoga also helps you stay fit, feel relaxed and be aware of your body. Sex, after all, is first and foremost a physical act.

Feeling chronically tired can also be a symptom of depression, as can a change in your sleeping patterns (sleeping more than usual, waking up early in the morning).

Depression affects not only your mind, emotions and body, but your whole life. See your doctor if you have several of these symptoms for more than a week:

- constantly feeling low and tired
- disturbed sleep pattern
- feeling isolated and worthless
- finding the smallest task impossible
- feeling generally stressed and anxious
- changed eating pattern, leading to weight gain or loss.

Should you have any thoughts of death or suicide, see your doctor immediately.

How to Say 'No' Nicely

Spare a thought for the one in your relationship who usually initiates sex. If it's not you, then you may at times feel positively pestered. Yet in some respects making the first move is quite a brave thing to do – because of the risk of rejection. No matter how long you've been together, nothing feels quite so galling as being turned down in bed, especially if you are really longing to make love.

So if you are the one who doesn't feel like it, make sure you let your partner know gently – and at an early stage in proceedings. Timing is important. 'Don't wait until the last moment and then push your partner away,' counsels Jane Hawksley.

The way you say it is important too. 'Try to say "no" in a loving, accepting way, so that it doesn't feel like a rejection,' says Jane Hawksley. 'Your partner only wants to make love when you do as well – that's what you really learn in a long-term relationship. What we really want is for our partners to want us. So try not to have a row. Just say, "look darling, shall we plan another time?"'

4. Being Bored in Bed

Desire is a contrary kind of feeling. Almost by definition, we want what we can't have and grow tired of it when it's freely available. In medieval times, eating salmon was a form of penance for monks in Ireland, because there was just so much of the stuff. Do anything often enough – no matter how much you enjoy doing it in the beginning – and sooner or later the pleasure will pall.

Denise is 39:

Much as I have always enjoyed sex with my partner, I do find it difficult to ring the changes. When we first got together we used to do it anywhere, anytime, but we simply don't have that drive any more, and besides, we seem to be permanently surrounded by teenagers who never go to bed.

So our options are limited these days. It has to be in the bedroom, and preferably late at night when their music is so loud they won't hear us anyway. I don't feel that I can tie him up, or get dressed up or do any of those raunchy things people do – just in case one of the kids barges in.

So there we are, getting undressed, socks, greying T-shirts. Hardly exciting. Into bed. Grope, kiss, a tweak on the nipples, bit of stroking, cunnilingus if I'm lucky, him on top – or sometimes me – and Bob's your uncle.

Yes, the earth moves, but not very far! And then next week, same thing all over again.

This is a central dilemma for long-term lovers. You want someone so much that you plan to spend the rest of your lives together; yet because you are together so much, there is a danger that you will stop wanting them.

The trick in long relationships, it seems, is not to rely on spontaneous desire. If you want exciting sex to happen, you have to *make it happen*. Forget all that romantic stuff about being 'swept away by passion'. All those raging torrents of desire tend to die down a bit once we are bonded into a regular pair. And besides, a lot of that is just about not having to take responsibility for sex – and so not having to feel guilty.

But once we have settled in a long-term relationship, we are allowed to have sex. We are *supposed* to have sex. We can't pretend any more that our desires are forces beyond our control. We have to acknowledge our desires, articulate them, act on them. Difficult stuff in a culture like ours that still believes at heart that it's a dirty business.

In long-term relationships, sex gets boring and/or infrequent if we just wait for it to happen. It gets better – much better – when we deliberately, consciously ask for it, think about it, plan it, work on it, revel in it.

COUPLE'S COUNSEL

So how do you keep sexual boredom at bay in a long-term relationship? One way is simply to stop making love for a while (perhaps there is a positive function of 'going off it' after all? *See Chapter 4*). When you start again, it could well feel marvellous, but as a strategy this has many risks.

There is, of course, lots of commercially available gear – from sex shops and catalogues – aimed at spicing things up. And if you fancy dressing up in leather, rubber or PVC, or if sex toys appeal to you, why not give it a whirl?

But your greatest weapon against getting stuck in a rut is your mind. Fantasy and role-playing can make things new again. So can an unexpected sexual suggestion. Or sharing those things you have never told anybody about what really turns you on. Or, better still, *doing* them.

For many of us, the idea of 'illicit' sex is very exciting. Having an affair; meeting someone new who will 'electrify' us; having sex in weird and wonderful places. Indeed, the most urgent, driven sex that most of us have ever experienced took place when we were teenagers – and all that heavy petting in secret was more fun than 'going all the way' turned out to be later on.

But rather than changing partners to have new experiences, why not try changing your experiences?

- Book into a hotel for an evening or more.
- Make 'obscene' phone calls to each other.
- Avoid the 'real thing' and go back to heavy petting.
- Get a babysitter to take the children out on Saturday morning – and go back to bed.
- Pretend you are having an affair.

LUST-BUILDERS

- Anticipation is the name of the game. The sexiest part of you is your mind, so use it to imagine what you are going to do later on.
- Lewd talk can up the ante beautifully. Make a phone call or send a note, spelling out exactly what you've got in mind…
- We all thrive on TLC, so smile, cuddle, say 'I love you' – and show a little tenderness.
- It's almost impossible to relax and concentrate on sex with your head full of work difficulties or problems with children, so *take time* to unwind from your daily routine before you get going.
- Enjoy a 'starter' – kissing, fondling, half-undressing – then stop and wait till later.
- A change of scene can work wonders in freshening up your flagging libido, so farm out the children and take yourselves off somewhere new. If you can't get away, find a new corner of the house – or garden – to give an edge to lovemaking.

- Obligation is a real passion-killer. There's nothing worse than feeling you've got to do it – yet again – when you don't really want to.

- Anger and resentment (about money, household chores, unkind remarks) will dampen any spark pretty effectively.

- Haste is a waste. It takes time, especially for women, to become fully aroused.

- Grabbing, squeezing too hard, pinching, biting: chances are that these will make your lover more petulant than passionate.

5. No Time to Make Love Any More...

Such are the pressures of modern living – combining work with family and social life – that sometimes it seems there is no time for something as apparently optional as our sex lives.

The facts speak eloquently for themselves: people in the West are working longer and longer hours, and the British have the longest working days in Europe. We also have the highest divorce rate. Not surprisingly, one of the things Relate counsellors notice about most relationships today is that couples don't get to spend enough good quality time with each other.

Mandy is 35; her husband Colin is 39:

We have three children and we both work, me part-time and him quite long hours. We are up before seven to get the kids off to school, then it's non-stop all day till we get home – via the supermarket – make supper and put our youngest to bed. I sometimes have work to do in the evenings too. Colin plays badminton one night, I do a step class another night and take my daughter swimming on Thursdays. We tend to go out with friends, or out for a meal or to a movie about once a week as well. That doesn't leave a lot of time for unwinding and having sex, does it?

COUPLE'S COUNSEL

We do seem to be busier than ever these days. However, do we have to cram our diaries quite so full? Is a meal out or a film 'more important' than sex – or are we making excuses, avoiding facing up to difficulties and resentments?

Hot Tips: Make Time and Space for Sex

- Put your television away – at least one night a week.
- Get a lock on the bedroom door – keep out the kids.
- Get out your diary and set a date…(if that seems a bit 'sad', remember that before settling into a long-term relationship you set aside time for sex too – when you 'went out' with someone).

FAMILIARITY BREEDS CONTEMPT

Sometimes it can be hard to get past the reality of your partner's day-to-day behaviour, especially if he or she is short on charm when he or she gets home from work. How do you make advances to someone who hasn't spoken to you for hours on end because he or she has brought so much work home? How do you look forward to seeing someone come in the door when you know you are going to get no more than a grunt for a greeting?

Jane Hawksley believes that many a relationship is made or broken in our ordinary domestic exchanges:

We all work far too hard these days and we pay the price in our relationships. Yet one small gesture – such as a smile – is so significant between a couple. That first 20 seconds when you meet at the end of the day is as important as the rest of the evening. So many couples destroy their relationship in that 20 seconds. If you come home into an atmosphere, both of you are going to suffer.

I've been counselling for 25 years and I've seen how a relationship can founder or carry on in no more than a split second. We operate at a very intuitive level. We know every little nuance of our partner's behaviour. We can all play the silent game, but someone has to take the first step to end it. Brainstorm those first 20 seconds; see what is the worst – and best – you can do with them. These are achievable, change-able things. Having made the changes, you can move on.

CHAPTER 6

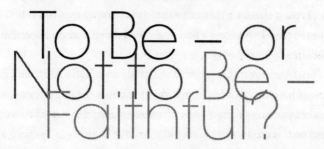

To Be – or Not to Be – Faithful?

Another way to deal with (or *not* deal with) trouble on the home front is to get involved with someone else. In a long-term relationship, chances are that at least one of you will be unfaithful at some point. The figures vary, but around 70 per cent of men and 60 per cent of women have affairs in the course of their marriage or partnership.

The reasons – and the results – are complex and varied, but one way or another, your relationship is bound to be affected.

Helen and Lisa are two women at opposite ends of the fidelity spectrum. Helen is 23 and feels that staying faithful to one partner is impossibly restrictive. Lisa is 38, has three children, and is very happily married to her first and only boyfriend:

Helen: 'The best of both worlds.'

'I've never been faithful to anyone, ever. I don't feel that human beings are designed to be with one person for the rest of their lives.

To me, it is a very bizarre concept. It goes back to that animal, territorial feeling that I can't bear to share everything; that is a threat to my autonomy. I also have a fear of settling down and thinking that I haven't really *lived*.

'Yet I thrive on the security of being in a relationship and I've been with my current boyfriend for six months. I have always gone straight from one relationship into another, and I have not had a day on my own since I was 15 years old.

'I was madly in love with my first boyfriend and we were together for a year and a half. But at the end of it he slept with someone else which totally destroyed me. We carried on together for a while, but then I slept with his friend as a kind of revenge. I found I could have the excitement of an illicit affair *as well as* the security of a long-term relationship. I had the best of both worlds.

'That's when I got my taste for having affairs. It is so easy to lie. I have very little conscience about it. If two people are attracted to each other and it's not hurting the other person – because he doesn't know about it – what's wrong with that? Nowadays I have affairs just for the hell of it. The sexual excitement of someone new only lasts for about a month, and men stop telling you that you're attractive after a short while. I wouldn't marry anyone I hadn't been unfaithful to, because having an affair is a test of the relationship.

'I want to be wanted by more than one person. I need to be validated by someone else. It's an insecurity thing; confident people aren't unfaithful. At university I was terribly unfaithful to my boyfriend. When you are in a steady relationship you don't usually get to hear that people fancy you, and you can feel completely left out. So when someone starts flirting with me I think – Wicked! They fancy me! – and I can't turn them down.

'I couldn't cope if my boyfriend had an affair. I do operate a double standard. But he's not the type to do that and I do completely trust him. If he so much as snogged his ex I would go mad.

'Nearly everyone I know is unfaithful. A lot of it is to do with alcohol; I've never done it sober. It's more exciting sexually – and it's fun!'

Lisa: 'It doesn't worry me that he is my only lover.'

'Patrick was my first boyfriend. We met when we were 16 and we were completely in love with each other. But sexually it wasn't a wild, passionate thing where we tore each other's clothes off in lust. I was a bit scared at first, and he hadn't slept with anyone else either, so we learned together. From then on we always wanted sex and we did it quite a lot. There has never been anyone else for either of us.

'It was three years before we got married. During that time he was away for a spell of six months and I had three other boyfriends while he was away, but I didn't have sex with any of them.

'It doesn't worry me that he has been my only lover. Sometimes I feel that perhaps I am a bit naive in having had only one man in my life, but sex is sex whoever you are with. I have very honest conversations with lots of my friends and I've concluded that I have a much better sex life than many of them.

'We both feel free to say what we want sexually. At the end of the day it's all about being pleased. A few years ago I discovered my G spot and sex got seriously good. On average we make love about twice a week, which I think is plenty.

'But Patrick is more physical and affectionate than I am. We went through a time when he wanted sex more than I did; when the children were small I just wanted a bit of space.

'He was worried that I didn't really love him. Now he realizes that I do love him, but there are times when I just don't want sex. I think it's really important to do it when I *want* to do it – and for him to know that. I've never once done it and not enjoyed it. He says – 'You *do* enjoy it; why don't we do it more often?' I've explained that, like most women, I have a lot of other demands upon me. I've never let him have sex just to please him and I've never faked an orgasm. He just has to keep going!

'Patrick is very romantic and makes a big effort to seduce me. We hardly ever make love in our bed; it's usually downstairs after the children have gone to sleep. He sets up candles and makes the environment right. He makes a big effort; he's really sweet.

'We've had our ups and downs and we've learned a lot together. He's travelled such a long way in realizing what women are. He's much happier since he's understood that I really do love him and fancy him.

'I'm absolutely madly in love with him at the moment and now is the best time yet for us sexually. I can't imagine myself ever being with anyone else. I haven't got a moral view and I wouldn't say 'I'd never do that'; I've just been very lucky so far. It's been 20 years and still I could cry after we make love; it's such a deep feeling.'

A Search for Happiness – or a Thirst for Disaster?

Most of us in long-term relationships are somewhere along this spectrum between Lisa's and Helen's experience. At times we've looked beyond our partners to find excitement, comfort or admiration. Some of us retreat again; some of us keep going; but by and large we all have to address certain key questions. Where should we draw the line between being faithful and unfaithful? Are we prepared to overstep that line? How much does it really matter – and can we deal with the consequences?

Depending on your personal beliefs, the experience of being unfaithful to your partner can involve a great deal heart-searching, crippling guilt or straightforward pleasure. But more often than not, there is potential for tremendous hurt, especially when children are involved. The novelist Tim Parks, writing in *The Independent* (21/9/96), tells the story of his friend 'Alistair' who longs to leave the claustrophobia of his marriage for the rejuvenation of an affair. Yet leaving his children is an impossible prospect:

All of us have so much potential that will never be realised within the confines necessary to weave anything together. As I think back on the many people I know who have divorced or separated or left each other and got back together, it occurs to me that while most of them talk earnestly of their search for happiness, their dream of the perfect relationship, what really drives them is a thirst for intensity, for some kind of destiny, which often means disaster...For many of us, and especially for men, who do not bear children and do not breastfeed them, the only thing that is immediately felt to be sacred, the only meaningful intensity, or the last illusion, is passion.

Alistair eventually loses his wife, his children and his lover.

But it doesn't have to be that way. Many people do manage to maintain intense and intimate friendships with potential lovers and/or ex-lovers without overstepping the mark – and without putting their long-term relationships at risk.

Sally is 40 and describes herself as 'very happily married':

I think it is a great mistake to expect everything from one person in life. The idea that you will meet Mr Right and from then on it's Happily Ever After is not just romantic rubbish, it's damaging rubbish. How can a relationship survive the years if you put such a burden on anyone? Of course our relationship is central, but I get a lot of fun and affection and support from other people.

I also have several other men in my life, men who I like and admire and am attracted to. They are mostly very old friends; some are old boyfriends, and when I get the chance we go out for a drink or meet for a meal. We have a laugh, we flirt, sometimes we hug or have a brief kiss – but we never actually 'do it'.

These relationships are important to me because they remind me that I am attractive, that maybe I do have other options should I ever want to take them up. That means I am not trapped in my relationship, but that I have positively chosen to stay with my partner.

Sexual monogamy, after all, is a strange ideal. The idea that we should commit ourselves to spending the rest of our lives with one individual, forswearing attraction to all others, may have made sense in a world where people didn't live much beyond 40 and needed to be sure that their property was passed on to their genetic offspring. But the world has changed.

Ironically, it is still in the western world where romantic love is the Holy Grail – and where the divorce rate is around 40 per cent – that people think of monogamy as 'right'. We tend to forget that millions of people in the rest of the world live in families where having two, three or four wives is the norm. (Women, alas, are rarely allowed the same luxury in taking their pick of lovers.)

And although we may love one person and wish to remain sexually faithful to that person, it does not mean that we have to deny our attraction – even love – for other people. Many women have emotionally intimate relationships with particular men whom they never sleep with.

Sometimes these are old lovers whom we can feel perfectly safe with because we have already exhausted all the possibilities. For some women, they are men we will never touch because what we value is their romantic distance. Rather like the days of courtly love when knights undertook heroic deeds for their unattainable lady loves, these male friends love us from a respectful distance. The very fact that we are not having sex with them keeps the relationship above the murky waters of pain and betrayal. In fact, a non-affair can be more romantic – and more long lasting – than any sexual liaison.

Beth is in her early 40s and has a non-lover who knows more about her than anyone else in the world, including her husband:

Although I've been married for 20 years and we've got two children, I have a chap who I'm very close to. Sixteen years ago we found ourselves having emotions that we shouldn't have. Whenever we saw each other we would drink half a bottle of whisky and talk until three in the morning, sharing confidences we don't share with anyone else.

On numerous occasions we have spent the night in the same bed, but we haven't had sex because we knew it would ruin our relationship. The minute we overstepped the boundary we risked ruining two families. Celibacy made our relationship special.

Then about six years ago we came very close to breaking our own rules – and we spent the next year avoiding each other. It took a long time to get over that, but now we are back where we were. My husband knows that we spend a long time on the phone to each other, but he doesn't know how often we speak and he doesn't need to know. It's our secret.

For Cheryl, it is an old flame who provides her with a special magic which she misses in her marriage:

I still see the man I had a long – but impossible – relationship with before I got married. I was completely burned out and frazzled by the time we split up. It was always a yo-yo relationship, up and down to the extremes, but I loved every minute of it. I used to cry when we had sex it was so wonderful.

After I left him I married a man who is like a rock. My marriage is a straight line; some people would say it was boring but in those nine years with my first love I was discovering what I really needed and I decided that the top of my list is emotional security.

The last time we had sex was nine years ago, before I got married, but I still love seeing him. We just share a couple of hours of sanctity together. These days we still have the magic but not the sex. My husband doesn't know; why should he?

By Any Other Name?

Emily has been married for nearly 30 years and has two grown-up children. She has recently fallen in love, but because her lover is a woman, her husband doesn't feel she has been unfaithful to him:

'We didn't marry for love; it was for appearances. I knew that I was gay even then, but because of my religious background, I thought it was sinful and I hoped marriage would keep a lid on all that. I embarked on marriage with the intention of being faithful and of "purifying" myself, and after seven years we had a child. I hoped that motherhood would be enough for me, and in some ways it was. But then I fell in love with a woman.

'I have told my husband and he accepts it. To him it doesn't seem like infidelity. He sees it as an unfulfilled part of me being sorted out. It would hurt him too much to say that I've always been gay, and so I haven't told him that. He is a good man; I just don't love him.

'I still have sex with him although, if I had the choice, I would not. For the sake of peace and quiet it carries on. It's not horrendous or coercive – he is a good man – but to end that would be too cruel to him. I used to feel that, in love, all should be pure and honourable, but I've found that life is not like that. I have sex with him because I feel it is what I owe him.

'I don't feel I am being unfaithful to him either, because unfaithfulness involves a lie. I have told him about my lover and so there is no deceit. He also sees that I am very, very happy. I am a transformed woman and much easier to get along with. At the moment it works, and I hope it's not hurting anyone too much.'

Jenny, aged 36, has made a clear decision to say no to extra-marital sex. The hazards, as she sees them, are too great:

I have had the opportunity to have an affair from time to time, but I decided I wouldn't risk it. It would have been too long distance, too infrequent – and I would run the risk of losing my best mate. My husband and I have a very strong friendship. We fight like cats and dogs at times, but he is still my best friend. I would have to go a long way to find someone who could replace him.

Anita, aged 40, has also decided to stay faithful, but not without regret:

I've been very faithful to my husband since we got married about 15 years ago, and unless we split up, I don't want to have sex with anyone else.

But I do feel sad that I'm not likely to experience that first rush of sexual passion ever again. When you're in a long-term relationship it's not a question of if you're ever going to have sex. You know that you are going to have sex sometimes; it's just a question of when. Not nearly so exciting!

In contrast, Lauren has surprised herself by having a brief – but exhilarating fling – with a man she met at a party:

I've had my best sex with men I haven't known or even particularly liked. I shocked myself at a party recently. My husband stayed at home with our three children and I went on my own. I found myself on the sofa with a man. I felt very attracted to him. I put my head on his shoulder and we started kissing.

Then I practically dragged him upstairs and had the most amazing sex with him. It was wonderful; I haven't had that feeling with my husband for ages. I didn't want emotion, just sex.

But at the same time I was thinking – here I am, someone in a secure relationship and the mother of three children, what am I doing? Of course I never told my husband. It would destroy him.

As Lauren acknowledges, infidelity is a high-risk game with emotional consequences which can last a lifetime.

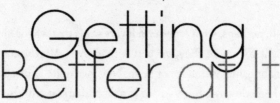

CHAPTER 7

Getting Better at It

Specialists in Each Other's Pleasure

There are great advantages to sex in a long-established relationship. What you may lose in spontaneity, you more than gain in deepening love and trust. What you lose in terms of novelty you more than gain in the deeper exploration of your sexual potential.

And while we hear a lot about the excitement of new romance, what is spoken about less often is the desire that a lover of many years can awaken – because no one else in the whole world knows you so intimately, no one else is such a specialist in your pleasure. With time, you and your partner have also grown in self-confidence, maturity and sexual expertise.

Why Long-term Lovers Have the Edge

Because they have more:

- experience
- mutual trust
- self-confidence
- specialist knowledge of each other's responses.

Quality Before Quantity

Above all, perhaps, what long-term lovers say is that when things are going right for them, they are better than ever. After years in the same relationship, you may not be making love quite as often as you did in the early days, but you are probably doing it with twice the imagination and expertise.

'Women get more naughty at forty.'

This was just one newspaper headline last year (9/11/97) as US-based sex expert Dr Theresa Crenshaw, known as one of the foremost pioneers of sexual medicine, revealed the results of a survey into sex and age. Dr Crenshaw found that, as women age, they become more orgasm driven, while men become more interested in touching and foreplay – and last longer during sex.

While Dr Crenshaw found that women in their 30s were ready to discard their inhibitions, telling their men what they needed to experience maximum pleasure, it was between the age of 40 and 50 that women really reached their sexual best.

According to Dr Crenshaw, this is the time when women have survived the demands of new careers and young children, emerging as leaders in bed, taking the initiative sexually and even seeking younger lovers if partners didn't fully satisfy them.

Louise has been married for 13 years and says that – despite occasional periods of relative inactivity – her sex life is now better than ever:

When we first married, if we got to the end of the week and we hadn't made love I would get really upset. But then we had children and we got used to a new phase of life; sex went out of the window. But when it came back in, it was very different. We don't make love quite so spontaneously any more. But we are much more deliberate. Much more inventive and varied and raunchy. Nowadays when we make love we start thinking about it in the morning, make hints about it all day, plan for it to happen in the evening – and take hours luxuriating in every aspect of it. Afterwards we lie around together talking, perfectly comfortable, feeling very satisfied with ourselves. That's a feeling that lasts for days and I know he is thinking about what we did and how good it was – and so am I!

Fiona, married for eight years, has also found that the tempo of lovemaking has changed – in many ways for the better:

The quantity of our sexual encounters may have diminished, but the quality has certainly increased. When we do it now, we do it good!

Since getting married only one thing has been added to my preferred sexual menu and that is that I enjoy the feeling of being caressed and cherished, especially after caring for three young children all day. So we have lots of lovely massage and I can just relish it all. If I am going to have sex at all it is to feel caressed. I do need him to slowly wind me down, which means I have to guide him a little bit – but this has improved the quality of our sex life greatly.

Orgasm: Improving with Age

The Janus Report, a US study into sexual behaviour, has found that although women have the most frequent sex before their mid-20s, only 39 per cent of this age group had orgasms 'often'.

However, 51 per cent of women aged 27–38 had plenty of orgasms, while 52 per cent of 39–50 year olds had a high orgasm rate.

(Source: 'Sex and Your Body'/*Cosmopolitan*, February 1997.)

This shift of focus from rapid, lust-driven coupling (as in the early days of relationships) to a more considered savouring of sensuousness marks out many a long-term lover. Candy has been married for 12 years:

We like massage and candles, a glass or two of wine and maybe some strawberries and a tub of really good ice cream. Every now and then we sit in bed and enjoy a touch of luxury, not for the children, just for us.

All this is not just a matter of technique, but of emotion – as Marcus put it in Chapter 1:

At the beginning of a relationship it is a matter of finding out about the other person. But you don't have that deep down feeling of knowing that your relationship really works. That comes with time and knowing what makes the relationship tick.

These days I am no longer thinking – where should I put my hand? What should I do next? We have got to the stage where we can forget about performance. Lovemaking has become less about technique; it is now more emotional and intuitive. It's about trust.

It takes many years of making love to get this sense of absolute confidence. It is about knowing someone very intimately.

And for all the excitement of falling into bed with someone new, there is also a tremendous amount of emotional risk involved. We are in many ways at our most vulnerable when making love, yet most of us embark on sexual relationships before we know our partners intimately – almost as a way of getting acquainted.

Three Qualities You Need for the Long Haul

I. EQUALITY

'Time was when he used to assume I would do most of the cooking and washing up and putting the kids to bed. We had big rows about that and if he wanted sex as well I felt it was just another way of using me. But he's changed a lot and these days we are far more equal. We both earn about the same amount and we will spend our evenings talking and doing various jobs together. The resentment has gone, and our sex life has really taken off too!'

2. EMPATHY

'I need him to spend time with me, talk to me, listen to me, pick up on his antennae just how I'm feeling. Then we are intimate; then we can make love.'

3. RECIPROCATION

'We went through a time a few years ago when he was out of work and I was supporting the family. Now it's his turn and I'm taking a back seat. It feels fair that way. We try to give each other the space and time we need to grow and develop; that way we stay close.'

With luck, and with love, our relationships survive but it can take many years before we really know that we are not going to be scorned, let down or rejected. Until then, sex may not be as good as it becomes later on.

'Confidence makes all the difference.'

For women especially, there is intense pressure in the early days of a relationship to conform to an ideal of what an attractive woman should be i.e. tall and slim with the face of a supermodel. It can take years before women relax into knowing that their partners love them for themselves, warts and all.

Mandy has been married for over a decade:

Our sex life is much better now after 10 years of marriage than it was at first. For me that's because I have a much greater sense of security, safety and familiarity with him after all these years. And because I have a better self-image now than when I was younger. Gaining more confidence in myself has made all the difference.

Not surprisingly, the quality of our sexual experiences is very much bound up with this issue of trust. Although some of us thoroughly enjoy casual sexual encounters, sex therapists say that women – and men – often report that they can't enjoy sex unless they feel 'safe' with their partners.

'Until my emotions were involved, my body said "no".'

After getting divorced at the age of 30, Jenny went through a five-year period of bedding every man she fancied – and there were quite a few. To her own disappointment, however, she found that no matter how keen she was to have sex, she couldn't reach orgasm. Not until she met someone she really trusted – and has since married – could she attain the pleasure and release she had been seeking all those years:

I had a good time in my years of 'freedom' and went to bed with more men than I care to think about now! But the weird thing was that I never entirely enjoyed it. Time and again I would end up in bed with an attractive man, full of lust and raring to go – but it would all fizzle out for me. Damp squibs each time.

Only when I fell in love with Paul – and only when I realized that he was equally serious about me – did the earth truly get moving again. Looking back I am sure that it was because I didn't know where I was with my casual lovers. It was purely a physical thing; my emotions weren't engaged – and without emotional commitment my body simply said 'no thank you'.

The Bottom Line

Whatever your situation in life, there is nothing like considering the alternatives to give you a healthy sense of perspective. Many of us imagine at times what life would be like if our long-term partner somehow painlessly vanished. Would we be free to find new love? Who would it be? What might he or she be like? Or would we live happily alone, doing just what we liked as the fancy took us?

But in the cold, clear light of day, when we think about yet another friend whose relationship has just hit the rocks, there is a sense of relief that we are still safely in calmer waters. Especially when we have children.

Caroline, married for 10 years, puts it like this:

Thank heavens I'm not single any more. All that pain and instability! It's a jungle out there, and to have to cope with that when you are older, fatter and saggier doesn't bear thinking about…

Half as Often – but Twice as Good!

It's a total myth that long-term couples give up on their sex lives – and that's official! According to the National Survey of Sexual Attitudes and Lifestyles, people in long-term relationships make love twice a week on average, compared to new lovers who tend to clock up three times a week.

The survey shows that heterosexual couples in long-term relationships do tend to have sex less often once they have passed the five-year mark. This is not at all surprising given the pressures of work, childcare and family which come with this kind of commitment.

If you are a pessimist you may see these figures and regret how sex diminishes with the years. But if you are an optimist, you will look at them and say – not bad!

- Men and women aged 25–34 in new relationships (under two years) said they had sex 12 times in a four-week period – or about three times a week.
- Those who had been with a partner for six or more years said they had sex 8 times (for women) or 9 times (for men) in a four-week period – or about twice a week.
- In the 35–44 age group, the 'new' couples clocked up 14 (for women) or 15 (for men) times a month. This settled down to the average of about twice a week after six or more years.

- In the age group up to 60 (the figures don't go any further), long-term couples are still making love on average once a week.

(Figures from *Sexual Behaviour in Britain; the National Survey of Sexual Attitudes and Lifestyles*, Penguin, 1994.)

Variety Performance

Another arena in which long-term lovers have the edge is in the knowledge that there's no hurry – and you've got nothing to prove. If one night you simply want to cuddle your hot water bottle, fine. If another night you want to tie him to the banisters and have your wicked way, fine also. You have already established that precious quality of trust, and so you are free to be yourself, to try new things out, be outrageous – or be asleep.

Hayley says her husband is her best friend, and after two decades of sharing virtually everything, she is entirely relaxed with him:

Because we have been together for so long – it's about 20 years – we are very comfortable with each other and we have had a complete range and breadth of sexual experience together in total safety.

We've had passionate, urgent sex. We've had falling asleep sex. We've had sex in the middle of the night and thought 'bloody hell!' And we've had a low-level kind of sex which we've decided to finish in the morning. It varies – and it doesn't matter.

Sue has the same kind of 'anything goes' relationship with her partner of many years:

What is nice is that with a long-term partner you can have that comfortable slow shag that might just peter out as you fall asleep – and then you can laugh about it in the morning. You can just do whatever you feel like doing; as long as it's between the two of you, anything goes.

Sometimes it's just easier to masturbate because you don't have to think about anyone else. Sometimes we are more lustful and we manage a quick shag before we go out.

Paula, who has been with her partner for 15 years, has a memory well stocked with sexual occasions to see her through lean times – and to inspire her when things get going again:

Depending on what is going on in our lives – with our children, our finances, our jobs, our parents – we can have some fantastic sex, or no sex at all. But because we have been together for so long, when I look at him I see him not just as my ageing bloke, but as the man who made love to me on the beach in Greece, on the train across Europe, and tied to the bedposts in a hotel in Spain.

No one else has those intimate memories; just us. No one else knows what he is capable of, what he smells like, tastes like, sounds like in sex. It's a bond so strong it's a bit like having children together; nothing can change the history of our intimacy and what we have made and shared. It's there, I can rely on it to sustain me – and I can conjure up images of us making love together any time I like.

'It's you I want – but you transcended…'

This extract from the diary of Rachel, who has been with her partner for 15 years, sheds light on how they manage to keep their relationship alive:

'We got a babysitter and went out for a drink last night. We started talking about sex and he said – tell me your fantasies then. I said I thought that women's fantasies were more emotional than men's; they were about being loved and made to feel special and wonderful.

'I also said I had fantasies about making love to certain Hollywood hunks, and that I bet he thought about fantasy women too. I wondered if long-term couples all over the country were not really making love to each other but to someone else in their minds?

'He said, no, I'd missed the point. What he wanted was me, but me transcended. Not the one who does the washing up or who wipes children's noses, but the one who gave him an image of backside bending over in suspenders all those years ago. What he said he wanted was not the kind of masturbatory images you get in porn mags – he thinks they are really boring – but specific sensory triggers.

'Just as crisp air and the smell of woodsmoke brings autumn powerfully to mind, he said, certain settings and scenarios can bring sexual pleasure powerfully to mind. It is about transcending the everyday to find the sexual in your partner.

Fun and Games

For many couples, too, trust and continuity bring opportunities to learn about sex by experimenting in their own pleasure:

Sally has been with her partner for 20 years:

When we first got together it was pure lust, no need for fore-play or getting in the mood; we were always in the mood. But after a few years that began to fade a little – and so we started to have fun with some of the optional extras. I found out that he really loves being spanked, and to my surprise, that it really excites me too. He is into rubber and some of the outfits you get from catalogues; those make me giggle but I don't mind giving anything a try.

Nowadays our sex life is like one long game of dressing up, acting out and playing roles. I've learned quite a few new tricks and so has he. When I was younger I wouldn't have dreamed of trying any of this stuff – it all had to be sheer romance and passion – but it's great. A whole new world of sensation and pleasure!

Alice met and fell in love with her husband when they were in their early 20s. It has been her first and only serious love affair:

We were very sexually inexperienced and shy when we first got together. But things have got steadily better between us as the years have passed. We're in our 50s now, and sex has never been so good!

Tony and his partner of 12 years have been trying out new ways of making love:

For years we only did straight sex. It was great, but it was totally lust driven, especially in the early days. Then a couple of years ago when we were staying in a friend's attic room, we discovered that we could see ourselves from the bed reflected in the glass of the skylight – if we kept the light on.

It was very erotic, like watching yourself take part in a porn movie, but without the guilt of feeling that someone is being exploited. So when we got home we set up some mirrors and watched ourselves again.

Since then we have been experimenting more – from sexy underwear and gadgets to a bit of mild S and M. Recently we talked about making a video of ourselves making love. We haven't done it yet, but just talking about it is quite exciting.

Hot Tips: Long-term Lovers Reveal What Turns Them On

'In a long-established relationship you have to make time for sex,' says psychosexual therapist Jane Hawksley. 'Get your diary out. Make a date to do it. It may feel cold blooded, but when you plan a meal, you think ahead about the details, you go to the shops, you plan it all. And the meal is much better for it. You can't snack on sex for the rest of your life.'

Anticipation is the name of the game. Let your lover know early in the day that it is going to be an evening to remember:

'One thing that particularly excites me is when he leaves me a note in my briefcase suggesting how we are going to have sex that evening – and where.'

Preparation helps you both to anticipate the delights ahead – and to make sure that you have the time and the space to make the most of each other:

'The knowledge that he is making a special effort can make all the difference. I sometimes find him upstairs setting up candles all around the bath. That gives me a great sense of anticipation and when we do have sex it is very exciting, almost as if it is for the first time.'

Ring the changes, surprise each other, get out of that rut. Boredom and routine are the great enemies of pleasure, so use your imagination and do it differently:

'Sometimes we go off to a hotel for a night. It helps a lot sexually to be in a different place, without the distractions of the usual home environment.'

Use your imagination. Whether you act out that scenario that really turns you on, or whether you just think about it, there is nothing like the gift of fantasy to help you see your partner through fresh eyes:

'I have my own private store of erotic images; situations I have read about, scenes I have seen in films, stories which have left me feeling all lustful. I can tune in to any of these while we are making love and transform myself – in my own mind – into all manner of multi-orgasmic harlots! Sometimes I tell him exactly what I am thinking about, and that really excites him at the same time.'

Practice Makes Perfect

Orgasm doesn't just happen when women have sex; it takes practice. One of the best ways to practise is masturbation. If a woman has no idea how to bring herself to a climax, how can her male partner work out how to do it?

Most boys learn to masturbate at an early age – the penis is more obvious and accessible than the clitoris – but girls often get the message that it's not on to touch themselves 'down there'. But if they never explore themselves it can take years to achieve orgasmic potential.

Which is a shame, not only because sex is fun and good for our health and wellbeing, but also because it helps maintain harmonious relationships.

Ms. Muscle: Making the Most of Your Assets

Well-toned pelvic floor muscles not only give men greater pleasure but can increase the intensity of women's orgasms too.

Pelvic floor exercises are designed to improve your bladder control and are usually recommended after childbirth. But keeping the P-C (pubococcygyeal) muscle in good shape not only gives women more control over their vaginal opening, but also improves sexual sensitivity and responsiveness by increasing blood flow to the area.

The muscle you need to exercise is the one you use to stop yourself peeing. Go through this routine whenever you remember, preferably three or four times a day – perhaps when you are cleaning your teeth or washing up or watching television:

1) Squeeze and release 20 times.
2) Contract and hold for three seconds, 10 times.
3) Repeat Step 1.

Not only will these exercises help you to avoid the incontinence problems experienced by a third of women over 60, but your sex life will greatly benefit as well!

Pulling the pelvic floor muscles upwards and inwards, tightening around your partner's penis, will enhance the sensitivity of your clitoris too, hastening the moment of orgasm.

Sensual Essentials

If you are into sensual massage with scented oils (and who wouldn't be?) why not try the 'sexy oil', ylang ylang? Aromatherapists say that this is a powerful aphrodisiac. Just add a few drops (but don't overdo it) to your usual massage oil and wait for ylang ylang to work its magic.

Clary sage is another essential oil reputed to have aphrodisiac powers – but this one is also deeply relaxing, so you might find that when your eyes close with pleasure, they stay closed…

Sexy Supplements

According to Lynne McTaggart, author of *What Doctors Don't Tell You (see Further Reading in Resources)*, at around the time of menopause women might find the following supplements helpful in maintaining libido:

- evening primrose oil (500 mg a day)
- vitamin E (400 units a day).

But she also points out that 'the most effective method of maintaining interest in sex and keeping the vaginal canal lubricated is to have regular sex'.

HERBAL HELP

Hypericum, a herbal treatment from the St John's Wort flower, has traditionally been used to treat depression. Recent trials have shown that it is as effective as current drug treatments for depression – with fewer side-effects. An added bonus of hypericum is that it improves libido in women around the time of menopause.

In a 1997 trial, 100 women between 45 and 65 were given hypericum. Before their treatment they reported that their greatest concern was their lack of sexual desire and low self-esteem.

According to Dr Barbara Grube, Medical Director of the Berlin Self Help Depression Group, who headed the study, 'the myth that sexuality is linked with youth means that many women feel uncertain of their self-worth during the climacteric (menopause). In addition, women frequently assume that, due to the changes in their hormones, they will no longer be able to find sex pleasurable during and after the menopause, and hence will lose their desire for it. However, it has been shown that human sexual experience is only loosely linked to the levels of hormones and their effects.'

After taking hypericum extract three times daily, more than 60 per cent of the women in the study said they felt sexy again and enjoyed or initiated sex with their partner.

After Children; a New Lease of Life

Another thing that time can do for our relationships is grow our children up a bit. After the wilderness years of early parenthood, the resurgence of desire can give a whole new lease of life to your relationship. No more babies waking up just as you get going; no more falling asleep as your head hits the pillow – and no more worries about pregnancy (whether you want to conceive or not).

Jan is just coming to the end of the toddler years – and reclaiming her identity as an independent sexual being:

When our two children were old enough to leave with my mum for the weekend, we took off and went to stay in a hotel, just the two of us. It was great, like taking off the 'parent glasses'. I felt 'he's a man', instead of 'he's a dad'. We had sex in the swimming pool and it was wonderful. I came home feeling like a sexual being again.

Small children have scant respect for your privacy, but some couples adapt and rise to the challenge of their changed circumstances by finding new ways – and new places – to make love. With mixed success sometimes, as Alison recently discovered:

We made love in the garden last week. Our son came out and caught us. 'What are you doing on the grass?' he asked us. We told him we were just looking for worms.

Moving on from the whole business of childbearing can also feel like a great liberation, as Vicky points out:

Since my last child I've been sterilized. And for us as a couple sexually, that has been the best thing I ever did. I've always been in control of my fertility. I've got pregnant when I wanted to and sex has always been a pleasure, not an effort. But now I no longer care what stage in my cycle I am at. Now it's totally spontaneous with no fumbling about for contraception.

And all being well, many women emerge from the years of birth and breastfeeding with a deep feeling of satisfaction. At the most fundamental level, motherhood can make us proud of ourselves and of our bodies which have nurtured and sustained new life. That earthy kind of confidence is very powerful and very sexy.

Nicky has had three children, ranging in age from five to 11, with her partner Mike:

Mike has seen me giving birth three times. What could be more intimate than that? He has seen how strong and determined I am; he has witnessed this miracle produced by my body. Of course there is a lot of mess, but – rather like having amazing sex – the urgency and passion of the occasion overwhelms everything else so that you are hardly aware of the gory details.

Having been through all that together, there is nothing left to feel shy about in bed. Having babies with Mike has given me immense confidence and liberated me from any inhibitions I might once have had about my body. As a result some of the best sex I've ever had has been since I've had my kids.

In short, long-term lovers enjoy a solidity and mutual strength that new lovers tend to lack. As a couple you have grown together. You know each other's likes and dislikes. You can be supportive, rather than critical, changing and adjusting to age. In the same way that we don't notice our children growing, long-term lovers don't notice their partners ageing.

Besides, age is the least of your concerns when you have already seen each other through thick and thin, family crises, births of children, deaths of friends and relatives, money worries, perhaps even the odd affair, and yet your relationship has survived.

Resources

Further Reading

Anand, Margo. *The Art of Sexual Ecstasy; the path of sacred sexuality for Western lovers*, Aquarian, 1989.

Bovey, Shelley. *The Empty Nest Syndrome*, Pandora, 1996.

Crenshaw, Dr. Theresa L. *Why We Love and Lust*, HarperCollins, 1996.

Hite, Shere. *The Hite Report on Love, Passion and Emotional Violence*, Optima, 1991.

McTaggart, Lynne. *What Doctors Don't Tell You*, Thorsons, 1996.

Melville, Arabella. *Light My Fire*, HarperCollins, 1995.

O'Connor, Dagmar. *How to make love to the same person for the rest of your life – and still love it*, Bantam Books, 1987.

Polhemus, Ted and Randall, Housk. *Rituals of Love; Sexual Experiments, Erotic Possibilities*, Picador, 1994.

Quilliam, Susan. *The Relate Guide to Staying Together*, Vermillion, 1995.

Rubin, Lillian B. *Intimate Strangers; men and women together*, Harper Perennial, 1990.

Swift, Rachel. *Women's Pleasure*, Pan Books, 1993.

Wellings, Kaye et al. *Sexual Behaviour in Britain; the national survey of sexual attitudes and lifestyles*, Penguin, 1994.

Helpful Organizations

The Amarant Trust, 11–13 Charterhouse Buildings, London ECIM 7AN. Tel. 0171–490 1644. For information on the menopause and HRT.

Marie Stopes Clinic, 108 Whitfield Street, London WIP 6BE. Tel. 0171–388 2585. Women's health check-ups, a self-referring menopause clinic and psychosexual counselling for both men and women.

Relate, Herbert Gray College, Little Church Street, Rugby, Warwickshire CV21 3AP. Tel. 01788 573241.

Wellbeing, 27 Sussex Place, Regent's Park, London NW1 4SP. Tel. 0171–262 5337.

Women's Health, 52–57 Featherstone Street, London ECIY 8RT. Tel. 0171–251 6333.